YES! YOGA HAS CURVES

DANA SMITH
THE YOGA DIVA

PHOTOGRAPHY BY: WANAKHAVI WAKHISI

ISBN 13: **978-0-69221-298-1**

This publication contains the opinions and ideas of the author and featured participants. It is intended to provide helpful informative information on the subject addressed in the publication. It is sold with the understanding that the publisher and featured participants are not engaged in rendering medical, health, or any other kind of professional services in the book. The reader should consult his or her medical, health, or other competent professional before adopting any of the suggestions in this book or drawing inferences from it.

For further information, or to arrange bulk sales or special discounts, please contact:

Spiritual Essence Yoga
(301) 574-3569
info@spiritualessenceyoga.com

Dedication

Thank you God for guiding me to my life purpose. It took many years and many lessons, but I am on the path and look forward to continuing for many years to come.

My dearest daughter, Brooke, you were the reason I opened myself up to another way of living. I will forever be grateful to you, my little muse.

To my husband, Eric, words cannot express how blessed I am to have you in my life. You encourage me to go out and learn as much as I can and give me loving reminders to walk my talk.

My darling son, Henry, your entrance into this world was a lesson in strength, patience, and letting go. Even though I am the mom, I learn so much from you each and every day.

To my dad, Henry, thank you for teaching me the way of an entrepreneur and a good work ethic.

To my mom, Joe Ann, thank you for teaching me how to work and maintain balance at home. Dad and Mom thank you both for your continued support of me. I look forward to the day when I can show you how grateful I am for the all the years you spent molding me into the woman I am today.

To my sisters Adrienne, Lisa, and Christina, thank you for putting up with my craziness as a youth. Our relationships have evolved wonderfully over the years, and I am honored to not only call you my sisters, but also my friends.

And to my dearest friend Sha-Ronda thank you for inspiring me, encouraging me, and holding me up for all of these years.

Acknowledgments

I would like to thank Wanakhavi for helping to bring my vision to a reality. You have such a gift, and you do your craft with such a humble nature. It was so easy working with you, and I am blessed to have you as a friend.

Thanks to all of the beautiful yoginis who traveled from near and far to lend their beauty to this effort.

Thanks to my SEY family who stepped in and helped keep things flowing at the studio.

Thanks to Manish Dalvi, our graphic artist, who was kind and patient as we worked in different time zones.

And thanks to our editor and fellow curvy yogini, Courtenay Brown. You came in divine time, and I was able to rest easy knowing you were working on bringing our stories out.

Contents

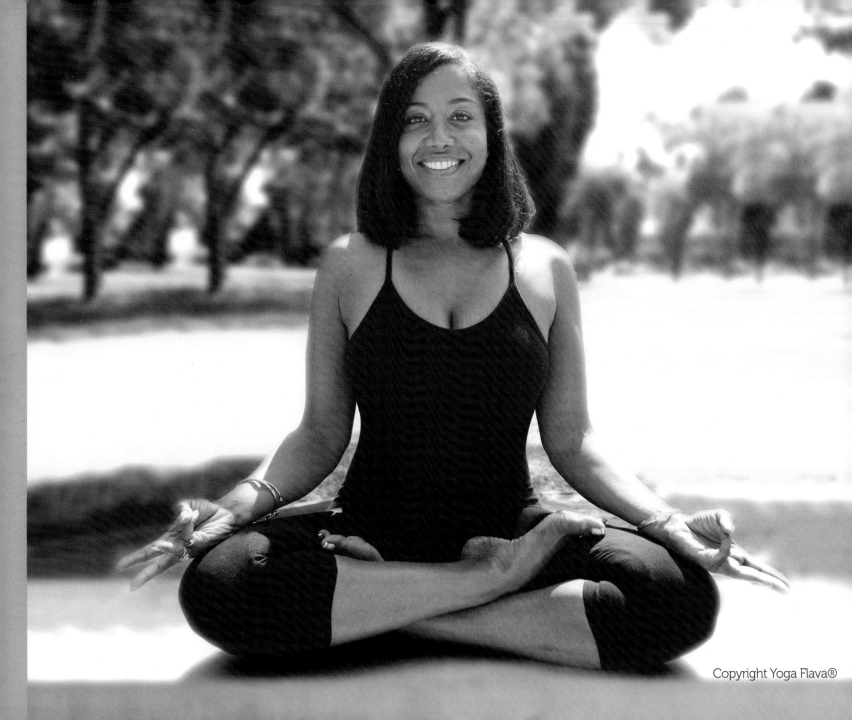

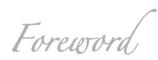

Foreword

Some people come to yoga to get a better body. In 1996, I came to yoga, because I desperately needed the tools to help me cope with the stress of my mother's battle with breast cancer. In the process, I learned that yoga means union with mind, body, and spirit.

In Los Angeles, yoga was beginning to gain attention for its healing benefits, so I decided to try it. After that first session, I immediately felt an enormous sense of relief. I wanted to deepen my understanding of yoga. The Center for Yoga offered a teacher training course. Although I did not want to become a teacher, I wanted to immerse myself in the practice and nurture my inner peace.

As part of the teacher training course, we had to practice teach. Once the course ended, my students did not want me to stop. I began to realize that it felt good to share the practice, and teaching kept me accountable to continue to grow and share.

In 1999, after my mother transitioned, I traveled to India to clarify my purpose in my practice. I understood that I needed to take the practice and interpret it for my people. Yoga "Flava" was born as a result of my journey. I realized that I was a part of a population that has evolved in a multicultural urban environment of which the sages of the past could not predict. Flava pronounced "Flay – vah" is a hip hop expression for contemporary style.

During this time, I also was going through a divorce. Once the divorce was finalized, and I turned 40,

I realized that I had gained a sense of fearlessness. So with the foundation of my studies, and my newfound freedom and fearlessness, I boldly represented my inner peace and released my **Yoga Flava for Relaxation** DVD in 2004.

At the time, I began to get a sense that despite my expertise to provide coping skills for stress relief, I did not have the visual appearance of what mainstream supported as a "yoga body." I'd been a "brick house" ever since the spring of 1976, when I turned 16 and my bra size went from an A cup to a DD!

Dana was one of the people that reached out to me with gratitude for representing a Yogini with curves. Her words of appreciation, gave me the reinforcement to "do me" – curves and all.

I am so proud of Dana for taking the initiative to create the movement Yes, Yoga Has Curves, and I totally support this book that is filled with images of curvy women that radiantly glow from an inner peace from their practice of yoga.

— **Robin Downes, Creator, Yoga Flava**

Ms. Downes is a 30-year veteran of the entertainment/multimedia business. She has an Emmy® Award for "Outstanding Individual Achievement in News and Documentary" with ABC NEWS "20/20" since 1981. She has been a certified Hatha Yoga Instructor and Wellness Coach since 1996. She is a syndicated original content provider and media personality to sites such as FeelRich.com and Elev8.com to name a few.

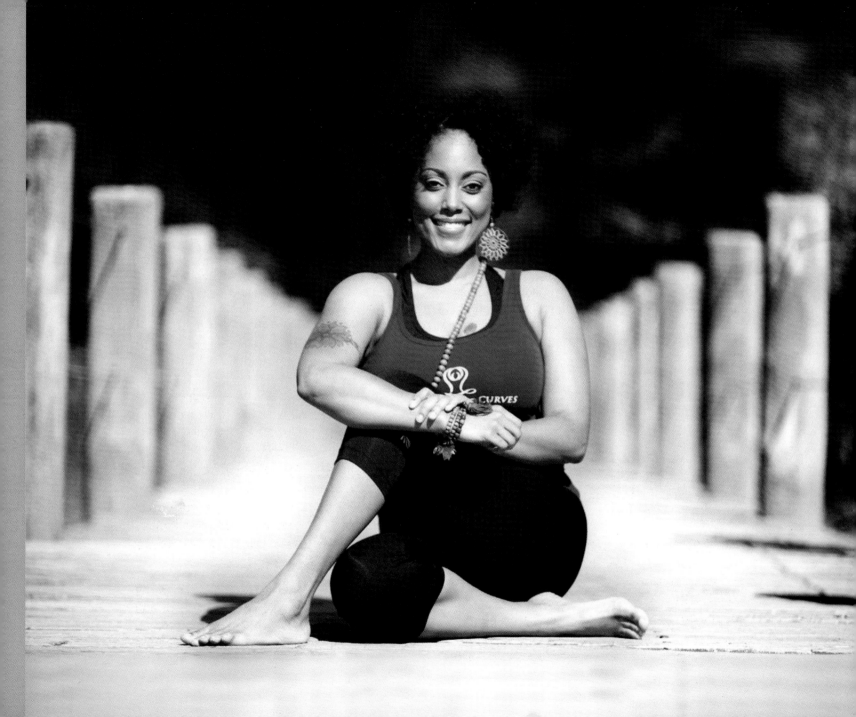

Introduction

I have always been very sensitive about my physical appearance. I was always the slimmest of my three sisters. My father's family has curves for days, while my mother's family members are tall and lean. I believed my mother's genes were dominant in me; so, I thought I would always be a perfectly effortless size 3. Well, reality hit like a ton of bricks during my first year of college, when I gained the dreaded "freshman 15," (which for me was more like the freshman 25). The change in lifestyle and lack of home cooked meals caused me to fill out.

At first, I didn't notice the weight gain, and nobody commented on it. But, when I went home for summer break, I realized that my body had undergone a drastic change. I'd filled out to a build that resembled my sisters. My family was supportive, and I actually felt good about my new figure. However, others were quick to give negative comments about my weight.

People would openly comment on my weight gain. They would even blatantly ask, "Is there something you want to tell me?" It wore me down. I forgot that I enjoyed this new me. I went on a mission to lose the weight. I subscribed to fitness magazines and watched countless hours of fitness television; but, I was discouraged by the body images I saw. Not

to mention, the body mass index measurements made it seem as if I was in worse health than I thought. I struggled to stay motivated and in the beginning it was hard to stick to anything.

Eventually, I got into a rhythm and began to lose weight by going to the gym regularly and being mindful of my diet. It took over two years for me to lose the weight. Being healthy made me happy and even though it was a journey, it was well worth the time. I broke up with my scale, looked at myself in the mirror, and fell in love with the woman looking back at me.

Even though I was happy with my body, deep down I felt like something was missing. Although I was physically healthy, I wasn't emotionally healthy. My mind was always racing, and I felt constantly stressed out. Despite my healthy lifestyle, I was often sick and I wasn't sleeping well. My doctor attributed it to stress, and advised that I take more time to be still instead of running around. Sitting still wasn't an option at the time, but I made a mental note to revisit it once the busy season ended.

A year passed and I was still in the midst of my busy season. I was searching for fulfillment and believed that I had to always be doing something in order to achieve it. In 2001, my busy season came to an abrupt halt when I became pregnant with my daughter. She was a wonderful surprise, and to this day I believe she was the answer to my prayers. The idea of motherhood terrified me, but I knew that I had to find a way to manage stress.

I was introduced to yoga by a coworker who practiced it to relieve the stress in her life. Initially, I was extremely resistant. I wasn't bendy; I wasn't as active because of my pregnancy; and I had no desire to put my foot behind my head (as I had seen in the magazines). But during my third trimester, 9/11 hit. I lost a loved one, and I didn't know how to deal with the stress, sadness, and anger I felt.

The tragedy also caused hidden fears to surface: I was afraid that I'd have to begin my health journey all over again, this time with an even bigger body. I was afraid that I wouldn't be a good mother. I was stressed out, and I needed help quickly; so, I finally took my coworker's advice, bought a few tapes and started practicing yoga at home. Even though I couldn't do many of the poses, practicing yoga helped me regain a sense of body acceptance and self-love. The unconditional love that I felt for that woman in the mirror grew even stronger than it was before.

Fast forward 11 years, and I have been blessed with another child, this time a very spirited son. Despite having had an emergency cesarean section, instead of the natural delivery we'd planned, I am 11 years wiser and I love my body even more. As I love it, it changes for the better each and every day. But what remains, what always remains, are these beautiful womanly curves.

This book has been a dream in the making for many, many years. The images we see of yoga do not provide a full representation of its practitioners. As a result, fuller-bodied, curvy women are hesitant to take up the practice because they don't think they have the "yoga body." I've been in one too many studios where instructors didn't know how to teach options for those with a little more "physical abundance," and I've heard one too many unyogic comments from both teachers and students downing voluptuous practitioners and doubting their ability to have a solid practice. This book is my testament that yoga is for EVERYbody and no one physical form stakes claim on the practice. The true essence of yoga is what you do from your heart, not what you do with your body.

This book celebrates beautiful goddesses of all curvy shapes and sizes and finally allows the beauty of our curves to be recognized in this blessed art called yoga.

Namaste'
Dana Smith, The Yoga Diva

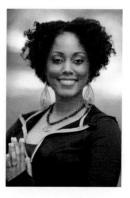

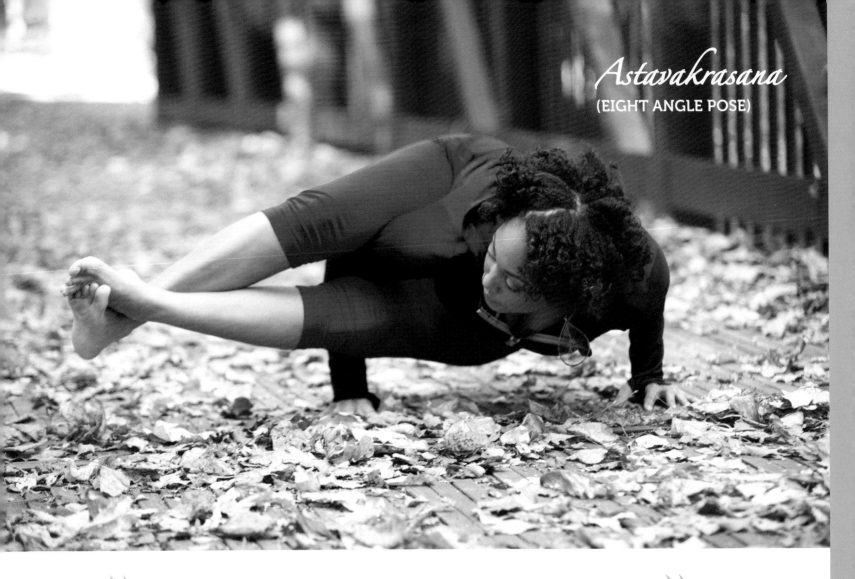

Astavakrasana
(EIGHT ANGLE POSE)

> The thing that is really hard, and really amazing, is giving up on being perfect and beginning the work of becoming yourself.
>
> **Anna Quindlen**

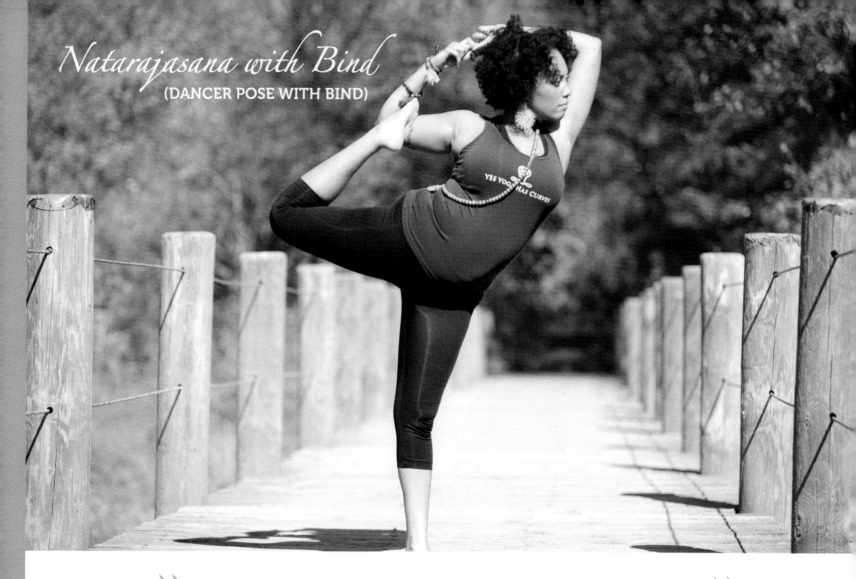

Natarajasana with Bind
(DANCER POSE WITH BIND)

> We delight in the beauty of the butterfly, but rarely admit the changes it has gone through to achieve that beauty.
>
> **Maya Angelou**

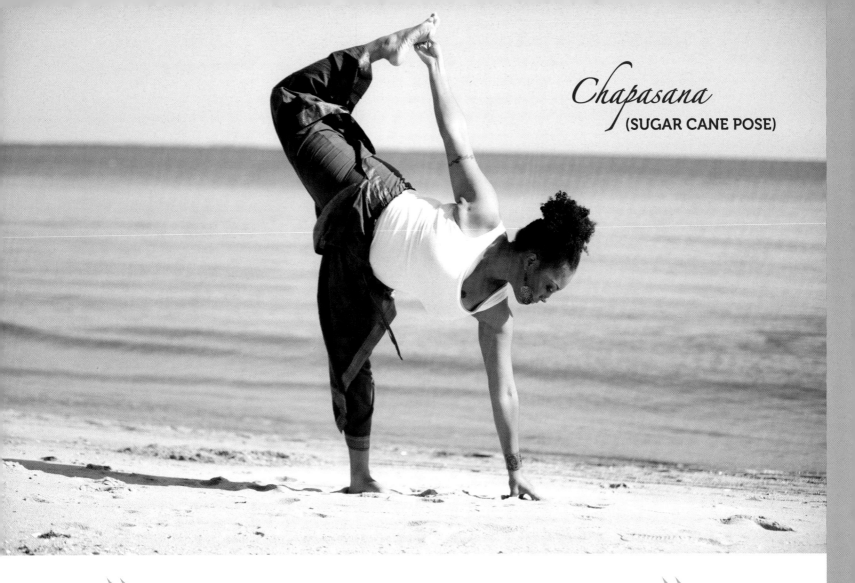

Chapasana
(SUGAR CANE POSE)

Self-compassion is simply giving the same kindness
to ourselves that we would give to others.

Christopher Germer

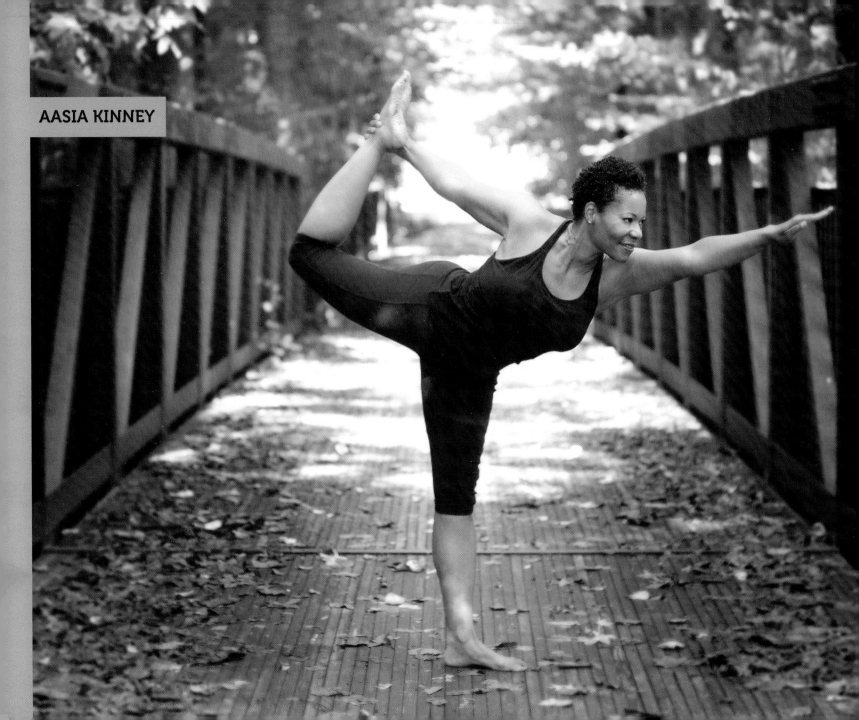

AASIA KINNEY

Be the change you wish to see in the world.
M. K. Gandhi

Natarajasana (LORD OF THE DANCE POSE)

Aasia's Story...

My yoga journey began three years ago. After a series of stressful events, I was in desperate need of peace and stillness in my life. Yoga helps me love and celebrate my body. It requires me to focus on me and my body by connecting in the mirror, with my thoughts, during Savasana.

Natarajasana is one of my favorite poses because it makes me feel powerful. It invokes my total concentration and makes me feel like I am a soaring high above the clouds.

The quote by **Gandhi** speaks to me because I finally get it. You can't change others. You can only change yourself. So, if something is not right, you have an opportunity to be the change.

I **love** my curves because they represent my femininity and my strength.

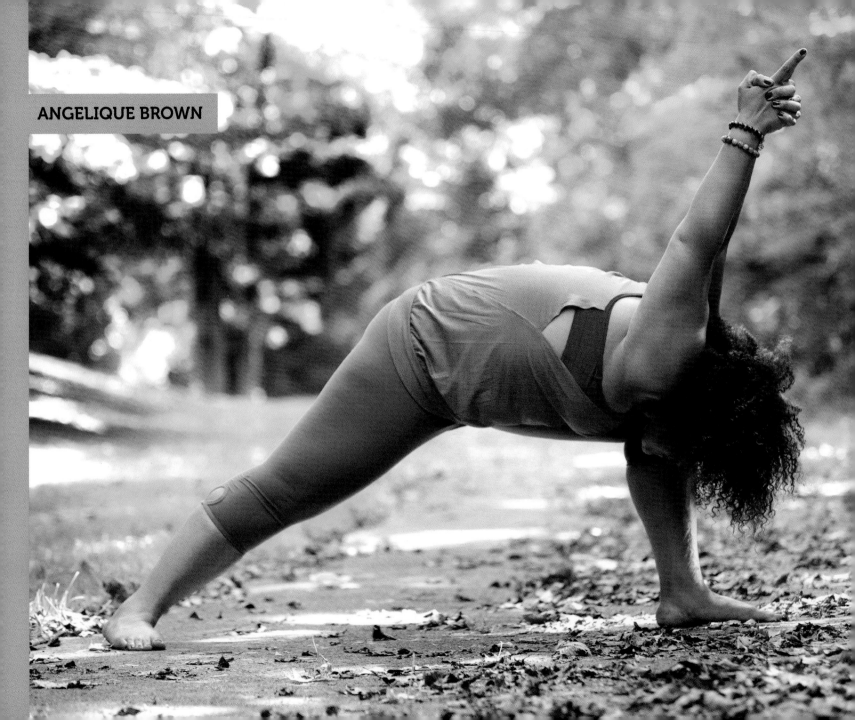

ANGELIQUE BROWN

Only by learning to live in harmony with our contradictions can you keep it all afloat.
Audre Lorde

Baddha Virabhadrasana (HUMBLE WARRIOR)

Angelique's Story...

I've been practicing yoga for almost five years. I started practicing as an alternative to my cardio and strength training programs. I was flexible when I was younger, and I wanted to regain some of my flexibility. Each time I'm on the mat, I have a chance to check in with myself and my body. There comes a point in each practice, when I forget about everything else and become connected to the pose. In that moment, I truly appreciate my body for what it allows me to do and how I feel in it. Yoga has made me more aware of when things are right and wrong within my body.

Baddha Virabhadrasana is one of my favorite yoga poses because it is all about opposing forces. I love the way that I have to use my legs to connect with the earth to stabilize myself, and how that grounding allows me to lift and stretch my arms. I also love that there's always a way to go deeper by widening the stance, lifting the arms, or even bowing the head. It feels like a wonderful offering.

The quote by **Audre Lorde** inspires me because I feel like I'm a ball of contradictions. But, I realized long ago that by denying myself things or forcing myself to give up aspects of my personality, I wasn't being true to myself. So now, I just accept me for what I am and allow the contradictions to just be.

I **love** my curves because they remind me of my femininity even in the most "masculine" of situations.

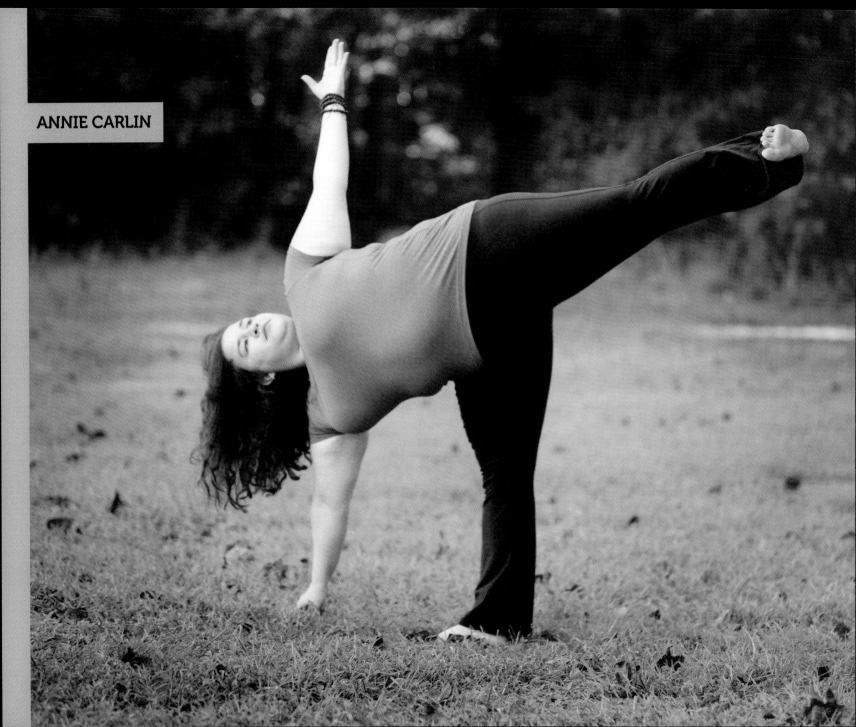

ANNIE CARLIN

> *Being firmly grounded in nonviolence creates atmosphere in which others can let go of their hostility.*
> **Patanjali's Yoga Sutra 2:35**

Ardha Chandrasana (HALF MOON)

Annie's Story...

I've been practicing yoga for over 11 years and teaching for almost 2 years. When I was in college, I was looking for something (anything) to relieve stress and find meaning in my life. I started practicing yoga at the suggestion of my roommate and fell head over heels in love.

When I began teaching, I discovered that my curves were my greatest asset. I had something to offer beyond the usual yoga teaching fare. I related to students and they related to me in ways I couldn't have imagined. Although my body has changed dramatically throughout my 11 years of practice, I've learned to celebrate my body in all its forms.

Ardha Chandrasana is one of my favorite yoga poses because there are so many ways to experience it. When I do the pose supported by a wall, I feel like I am flying!

Patanjali's Sutra brings to mind ahimsa or non-violence, non-harming towards myself. If I treat myself with love and joy, then others will hopefully follow. By setting an example of nonviolence/non-hate towards myself, I hope to inspire others to end their negative relationship with themselves and/or their bodies.

I **love** my curves because they are part of me. My body is my oldest, most loyal friend and strongest support system.

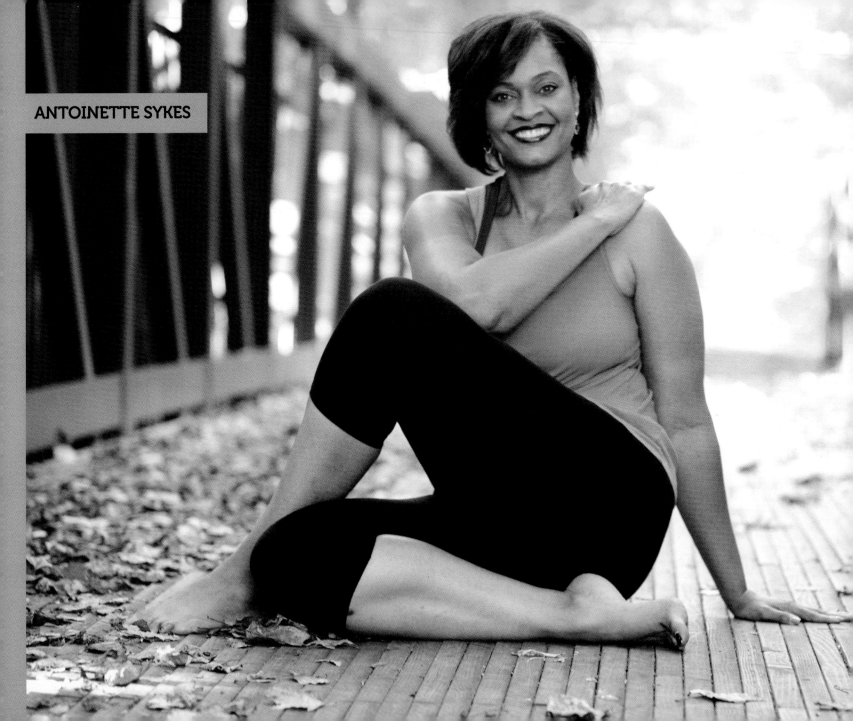
ANTOINETTE SYKES

Ardha Matsyendrasana (HALF LORD OF THE FISHES)

Antoinette's Story...

Yoga came into my life five years ago when I took my first Bikram yoga class. Hot, hot, baby! The sweat, the poses, the challenges, all felt so empowering and yet, peaceful. As an avid gym-goer, yoga seemed less stressful on my body, but it has been extremely powerful for my body and mind.

Ardha Matsyendrasana is a truly challenging pose. Practicing this pose gives me a deep feeling of accomplishment. It helps me focus on breathing deeply from my rib cage. It stirs my digestive system to know that anything unloving therein will be wrung out. It opens my hips to welcome more physical activity in my workout routine. My confidence simply soars when I come into the pose. I feel myself embody "Half Lord of the Fishes" navigating the waters of life and extending that powerful flow into every area of my life.

Yoga helps me be aware of my curves and simply just "be" with my curves. Yoga raises my body awareness and realigns me. It reminds me that I'm more than my body. Yoga is a loving experience. With yoga we can just do it. It's for you and no one else. Curvy yoginis a can utilize the strength of their curvy body and bend into something wonderful that only your soul recognizes.

Rumi's quote reminds me that everything I need is already within me. I need only stake the claim. My bread basket is fragrant, warm, and overflowing. As a result, my outside circumstances adhere to my Kingdom within.

I **love** my curves because my curves round out my soft, yet strong spirit.

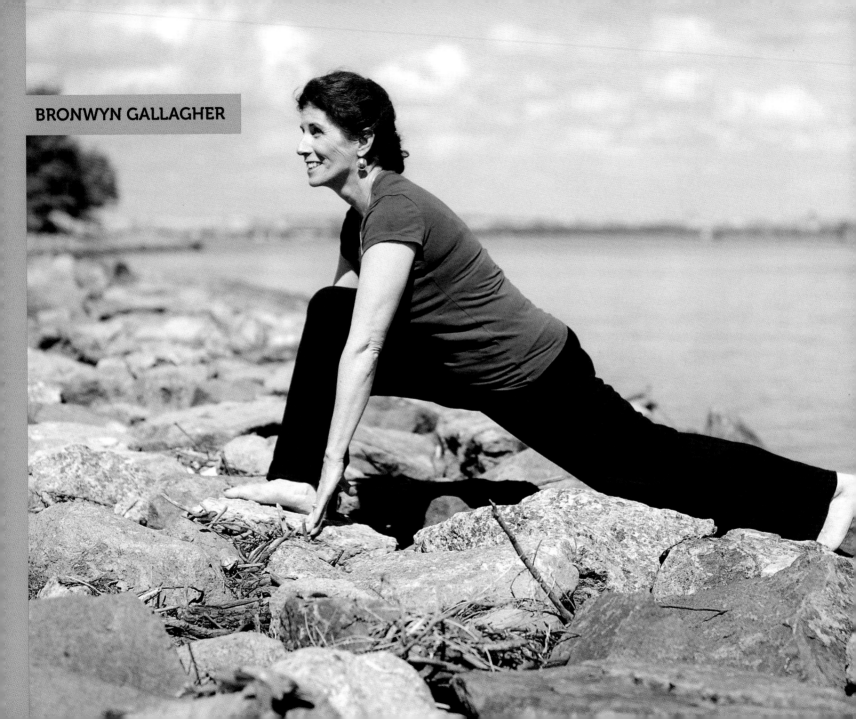

BRONWYN GALLAGHER

> What lies behind us and what lies before us are tiny matters compare to what lies within us.
> **Ralph Waldo Emerson**

Anjaneyasana (LOW LUNGE)

Bronwyn's Story...

I've been practicing yoga for 10 years. I was inspired to start practicing for the emotional, spiritual, and physical benefits yoga can invoke. Yoga helps me celebrate and love my curves. I have gained a deeper appreciation for my body and what it can do.

Anjaneyasana is my favorite pose, because I feel strong, powerful, and grounded when I am in the pose.

I encourage curvy women who are new to yoga to start slowly, be patient, and be consistent. Your yoga practice should not be a contest with someone else; it is a personal, individual experience.

Yoga helps see that message in **Emerson's** quote. Yoga helps me bring what's deep inside of me out. It takes a lot of patience. It reminds me to go deeper and to be brave enough to search beyond the surface to tap into my own abundant, inner font of potential.

I **love** my curves because they remind me that I am a woman.

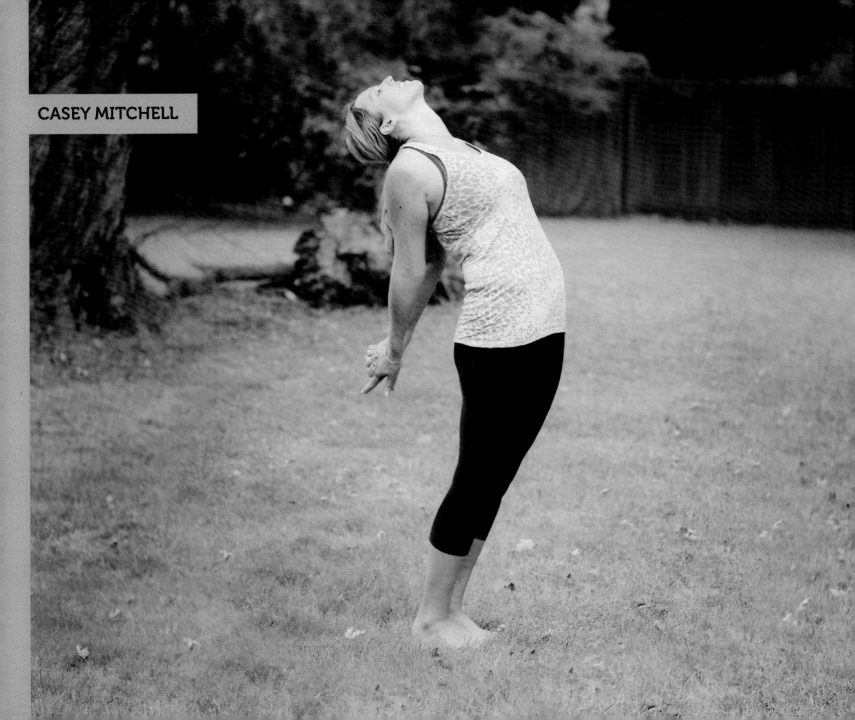

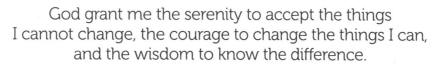

> God grant me the serenity to accept the things
> I cannot change, the courage to change the things I can,
> and the wisdom to know the difference.
> **Reinhold Niebuhr**

Urdhva Hastasana (UPWARD SALUTE)

Casey's Story...

I began practicing yoga in 2008, when a good friend suggested I try it with her. I fell in love with yoga immediately. I always feel so much more at ease after class. I have a history of hip problems, and I'm often frustrated when trying to reach or maintain a pose. However, I find such relief within my hips after I practice.

Urdhva Hastasana is one of my favorite poses because it reminds me that my life is part of a larger plan, a plan much greater than I may realize. In this pose, I can trust that my needs will be met. The pose also reminds me to reset and recharge after any challenge.

I chose the **Serenity Prayer** as my quote, because it keeps me balanced and focused.

I **love** my curves because they make me feel like a strong woman. I celebrate them and am thankful.

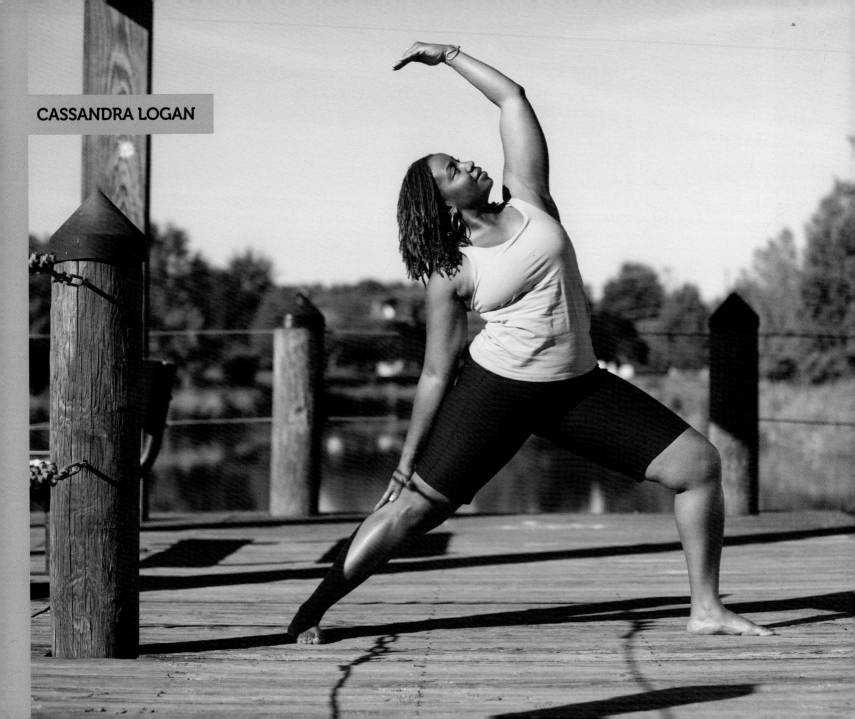

CASSANDRA LOGAN

> This above all: to thine own self be true.
> **Hamlet, Shakespeare**

Viparita Virabhadrasana (REVOLVED WARRIOR)

Cassandra's Story...

Yoga came into my life over a year ago, when I strained my groin. My doctor and physical therapist recommended that I start practicing to help heal from my injury. I love what I'm able to do today, compared to when I first started practicing yoga. My body has become strong and more flexible.

Viparita Virabhadrasana is one of my favorite poses because it exemplifies power and strength. There is another dimension to this pose. Being in the pose, as expected, makes you feel grounded and strong, but by opening your chest and reaching upward, the pose also embodies a certain grace and beauty.

Shakespeare's quote inspires me because it reminds me that no matter what, I should always be true to myself.

I **love** my curves because they make me look and feel strong and sexy.

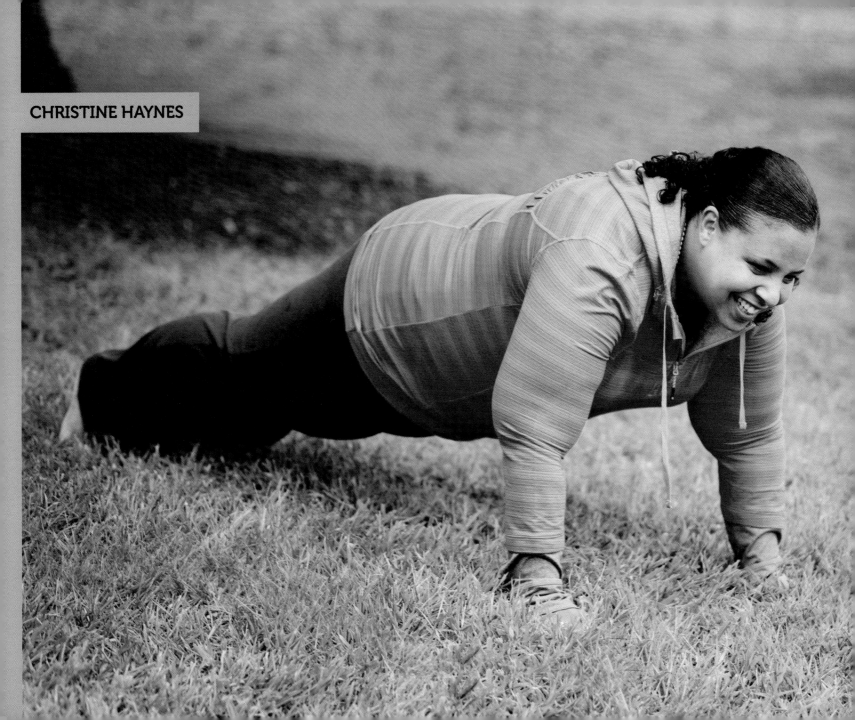

CHRISTINE HAYNES

> Our deepest fear is not that we are inadequate.
> Our deepest fear is that we are powerful beyond measure.
> **Marianne Williamson**

Phalakhasana (PLANK POSE)

Christine's Story...

I've been practicing yoga for about a year as a result of a knee injury. I needed a gentler form of movement. I had been thinking about trying yoga for some time. I thought it might be a good addition to my health and wellness regimen.

Practicing yoga makes me feel graceful (a word I'd never used to describe myself before I started practicing) and fully self-aware. **Phalakhasana** is one of my favorite poses because it makes me feel powerful! **Marianne Williamson**'s quote reminds me to SHINE!

I **love** my curves because they help me to finally appreciate the beauty and power of my body. I recently lost 70 lbs. Since beginning my health and wellness journey, I've found something new to love about my body every day. It's really quite remarkable—this vessel that was created for me holds so much power, mystery, and magic.

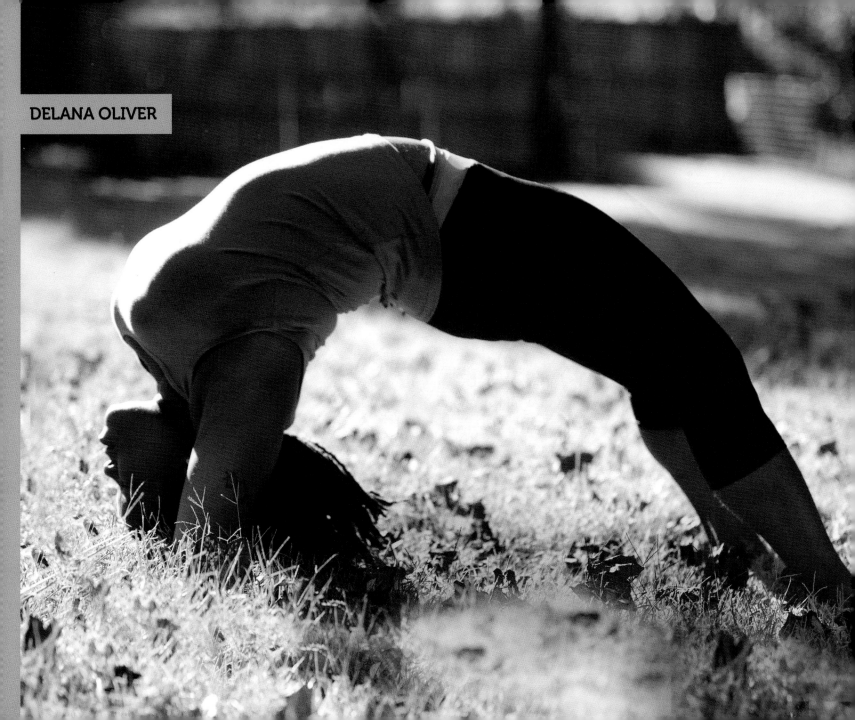

DELANA OLIVER

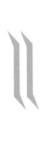

You have to let it all go; fear, doubt, disbelief.
Free your mind. The body cannot live without the mind.
Morpheus, The Matrix

Dwi Pada Viparita Dandasana (TWO LEGGED INVERTED STAFF)

Delana's Story...

I started practicing yoga nine years ago to compliment my martial arts training. It has turned into so much more than cross training over the years. When I come to the mat, I am free from judgment. I practice with a clear mind and enjoy the movement as I am in that moment.

Dwi Pada Viparita Dandasana is one of my favorite poses because it makes me feel uplifted and free. It encourages me to open myself to new possibilities and not be afraid of vulnerability. This pose says to me "press forward."

The **Matrix** quote reminds me that I have the power to release myself from my own suffering. Freedom starts in the mind and all else follows.

I **love** my curves because they represent femininity and in a way, they give me pride.

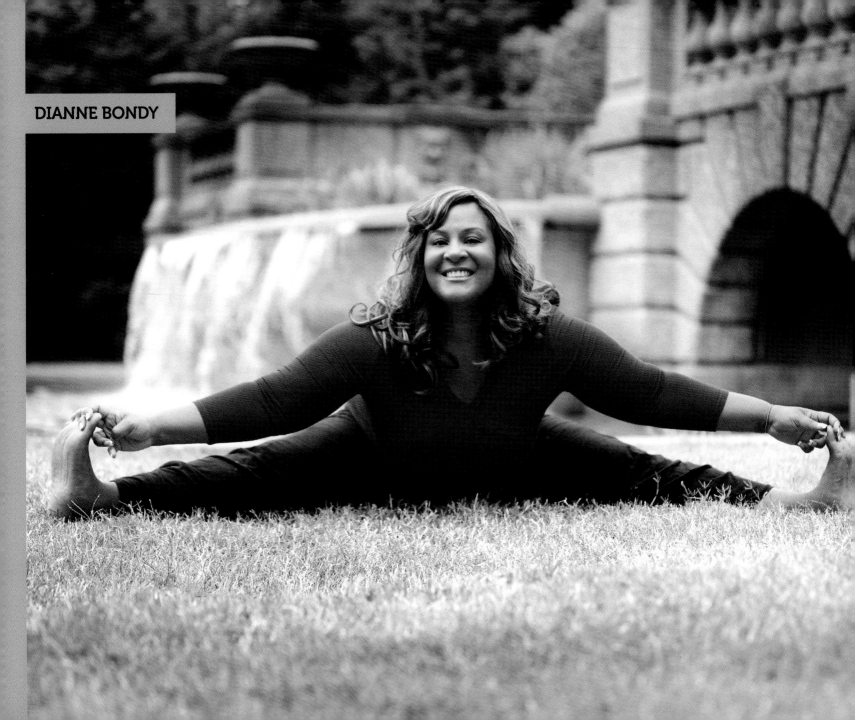

DIANNE BONDY

> Everybody can be great...because anybody can serve. You don't have to have a college degree to serve. You don't have to make your subject and verb agree to serve. You only need a heart full of grace. A soul generated by love.
>
> **Martin Luther King Jr.**

Upavistha Konasana (WIDE ANGLE FORWARD FOLD)

Dianne's Story...

I've been practicing yoga for most of my life. My mom was a yogini and we would practice together in our basement when I was younger. My mom had three small children under the age of four. She didn't drive, so she practiced yoga at home. I loved practicing with her while my siblings were napping.

Yoga is the one thing I have always done. When I practice yoga, I feel really free and joyful. It doesn't matter who is around, or what I look like. When I practice, I feel myself connecting with the Divine. Although I have drifted in and out of yoga, I always come back to my practice. I decided 10 years ago to get more serious about my practice and use yoga to serve my community.

I owned a studio for a while, and I loved it; but, I wanted to offer more than just in-studio classes. So, I started Yogasteya.com, an online studio devoted to yoga and diversity. I was really discouraged and tired of seeing only a certain demographic advertised and marketed to in mainstream yoga. No one was inviting the rest of us to join the revolution, so I invited myself and started my online site to feature all body types and cultures teaching and practicing yoga. I wanted to change what we see in media and on the mat.

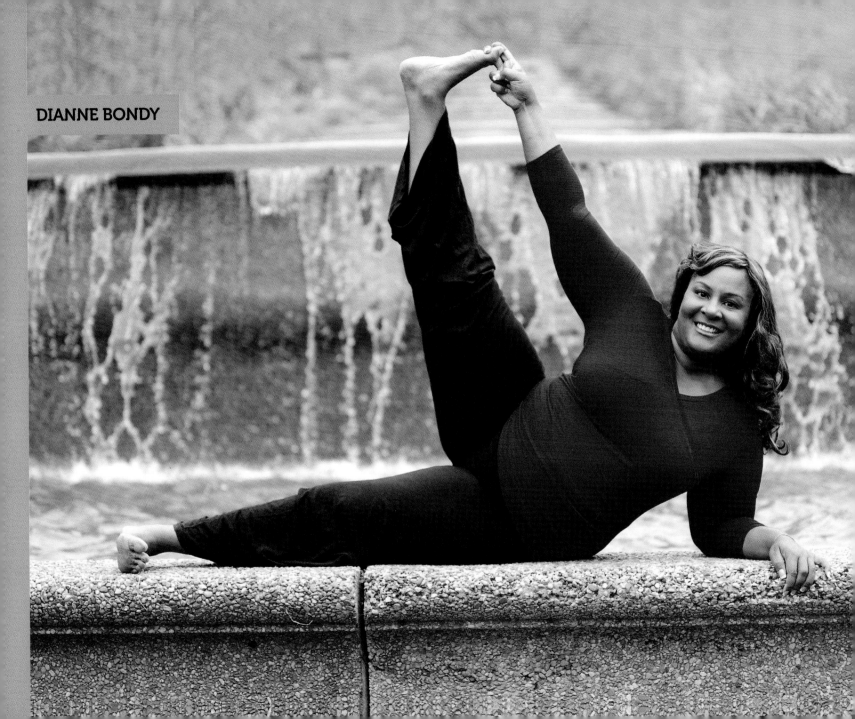

DIANNE BONDY

> Yoga should not be defined by your physical appearance or abilities. Yoga is in all of us and for all of us.
> **Dianne Bondy**

Anantasana (SIDE RECLINING LEG LIFT)

My inspirations are people like Anna Guest Jelley of CurvyYoga.com and Tina Veer of Yoga for Round Bodies. I have learned so much from these amazing yoginis. I am also inspired by people like Dana Smith, who are showing the world what yoga can do and what yoga really looks like.

Upavistha Konasana and **Anantasana** are two of my most favorite poses. I discovered Upavistha Konasana when I needed relief from lower back pain and tight hamstrings. The asana soothes my back and opens me up spiritually. I feel very strong and flexible in this pose. Anantasana makes me feel playful and beautiful.

I chose the **Dr. King** quote because it is so true and quite often forgotten. We all are great and we all can serve in beautiful ways.

I **love** my curves because they are a part of me. I love my curves because I love myself.

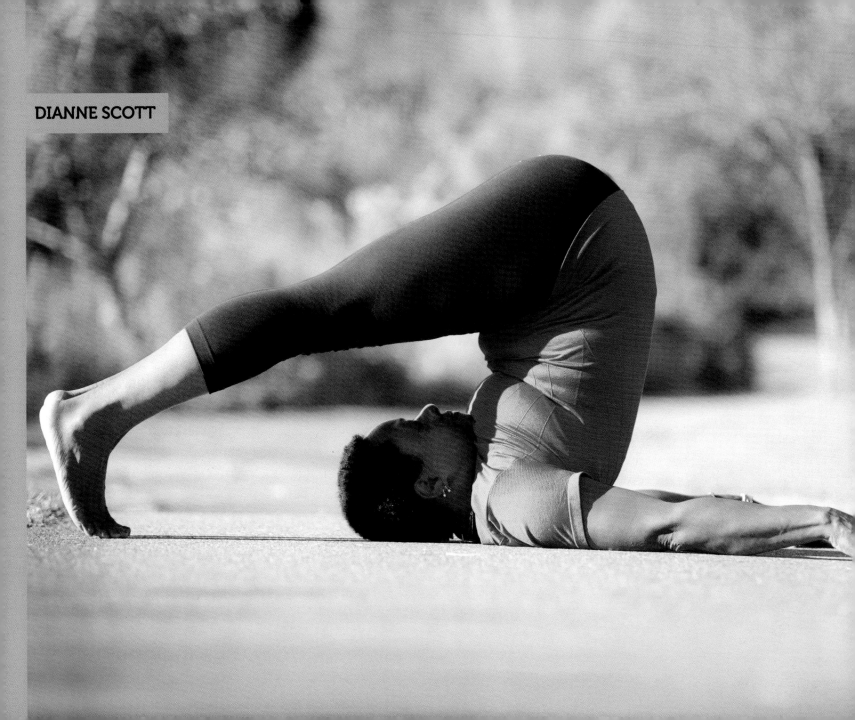

> *The first time someone shows you who they are, believe them.*
> **Maya Angelou**

Halasana (PLOW POSE)

Dianne's Story...

My first experience with yoga happened 18 years ago. I was a dancer at the time. Yoga gave me an opportunity to do something just for me, and not for the greater good of an ensemble. I enjoyed the freedom and anonymity of being... me.

Yoga has helped me embrace the changes my body has undergone as I mature as a woman. At 60, I realize I am no longer the same dress size as in my younger years, but I love my new womanly parts.

Halasana is one of my favorite poses because it invites me to feel calm and energized at the same time. Being inverted, my thoughts move inward; I feel connected to my spirit. While stretching my entire spine with my hips in line with my shoulders, I feel courage and strength. I love the dichotomy of feeling peace and vitality simultaneously.

This is my favorite quote from **Maya Angelou** because I have had a tendency to try to ignore the truth about a person and see what I want to see.

I **love** my curves because they make me feel more like a woman than ever before.

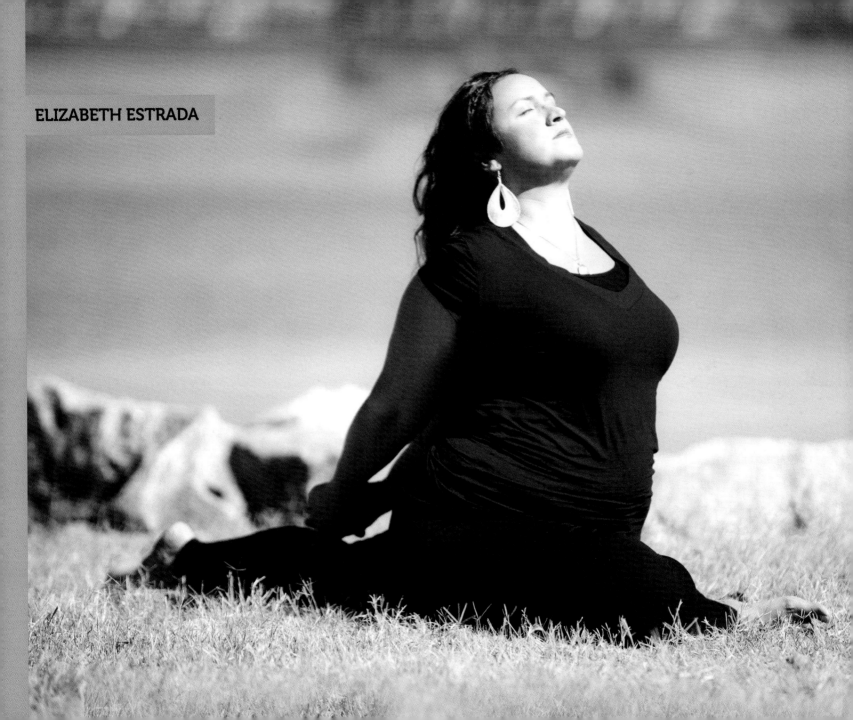

ELIZABETH ESTRADA

> I call upon you to draw from the depths of your being — to prove that we are a human race, to prove that our love outweighs our need to hate, that our compassion is more compelling than our need to blame.
>
> **Elizabeth Taylor (Author)**

Eka Pada Rajakapotasana (ONE LEGGED PIGEON)

Elizabeth's Story...

I was exposed to yoga teachings and yoga books at a young age by my mother. In 2004, after giving birth to my daughter, I began taking yoga classes on my college campus. My yoga instructor inspired me to practice on my own and dive deeper into the study of the self, an enlightened path and the eight limbs of yoga.

Every time I come to the mat, I discover new things about my body. The asana practice of yoga has given me a greater awareness of my strengths and weaknesses, and revealed areas of tension and freedom in my body. Yoga has taught me how to love all of these qualities as they are and to breathe with them. Yoga helped me find presence and stillness in my body. As a result of my practice, I am able to enjoy all my accomplishments and embrace my trials on the mat and off.

Eka Pada Rajakapotasana is one of the most often prescribed hip openers. Tight hips can be a contributing factor to lower back pain and knee problems. This pose stretches the outer hip and groin of the forward leg and the hip flexors of the rear leg. I have a different experience every time I practice this pose.

It is important to take your time with this pose and practice many preparatory poses as it does not always come easily. I enjoy the modified version of the pose because it allows me to engage my core and leg strength and express my hip flexor, hamstring and spinal flexibility. It's also a shoulder opening pose. Practicing the pose reminds me that I can take my sense of strength, flexibility, confidence, centeredness, and courage off the mat into everyday life. The feelings I associate with Eka Pada Rajakapotasana are exultation, joyfulness, surrender, and magnificence.

For me the quote reminds me that we, as humans, have a capacity to grow. We can find the inner strength to unite despite our differences. It is by our own free will and choice that we inspire hope and create a more peaceful future for ourselves.

I **love** my curves because they help me celebrate the voluptuousness of my body.

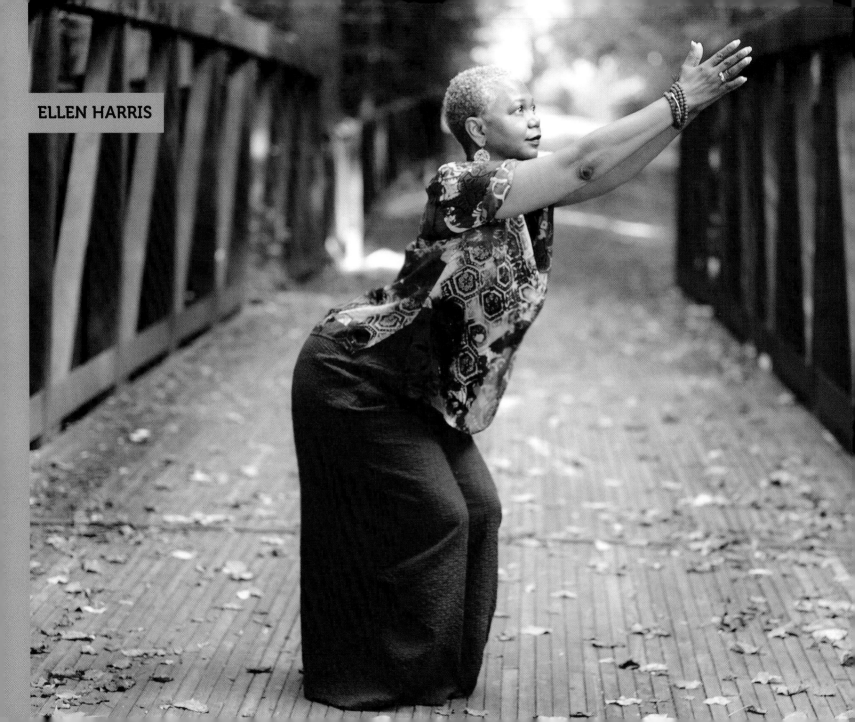

ELLEN HARRIS

> The spirit is power, the life that is in everything.
>
> **Unknown**

Utkatasana (CHAIR POSE)

Ellen's Story...

I have been practicing yoga off and on since I was in college. I was initially inspired to practice yoga to improve my fitness and flexibility. In June 2010, I was diagnosed with breast cancer. Luckily, I was diagnosed in the very early stages; but, I still had to undergo two lumpectomy surgeries followed by six weeks of daily radiation therapy.

My physician suggested some of the holistic treatments offered by the Breast Care Center, which led me back to my yoga practice and much more. I became a certified yoga teacher, Reiki practitioner, and a Thai Yoga Massage practitioner.

My favorite inspirational quote has no author and is described as an African oral tradition. I see my yoga practice through this quote because yoga lifts my spirit and enhances my spiritual power, which strengthens my life force and makes me smile.

Utkatasana is one of my favorite poses because it makes me feel balanced and centered. My feet are planted, legs and thighs are strong, core feels good, and my arms extend upwards with purpose. Practicing this pose has helped me in practicing various versions of **Parivrtta Utkatasana** and **Garudasana**. I've been able to grow from what I viewed as a simple squat to more complicated, twisting moves that invigorate my entire body.

I **love** my curves because they are a natural part of me, a woman of African descent with the hips to show it!

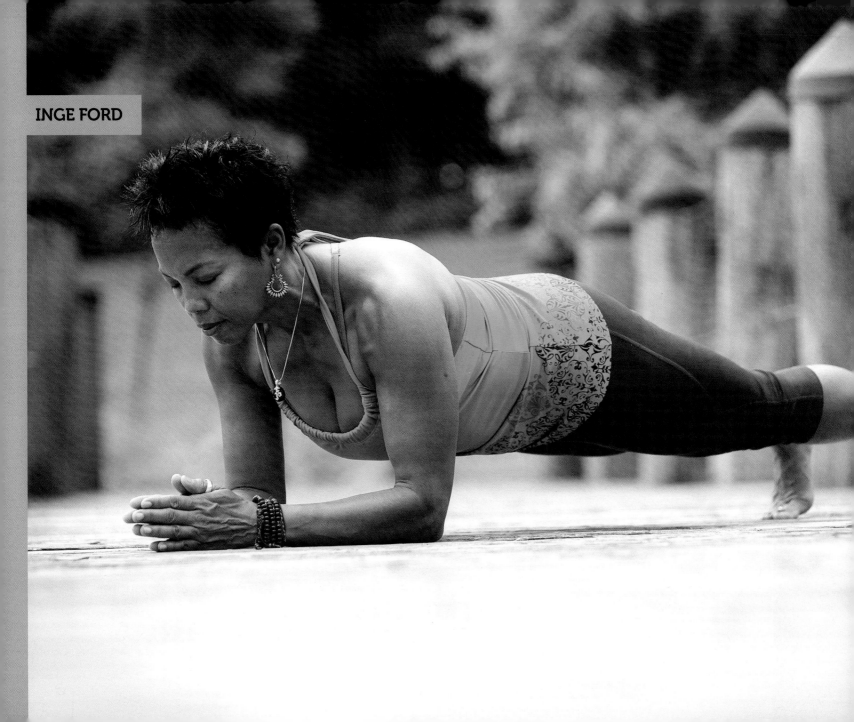

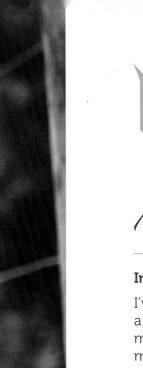

> It is not because things are difficult that we do not dare;
> it is because we do not dare that they are difficult.
> **Seneca**

Makara Adho Mukha Svanasana (DOLPHIN PLANK)

Inge's Story...

I've been practicing yoga for more than 35 years and teaching for about 4 years. I wanted to find a system that I could practice anywhere, anytime, with or without others and that would integrate my total being. Physical yoga asana complements my body type by opening and stretching my inner being. Feeling stronger internally affords me more calm, acceptance, confidence and gratitude of my sturdy frame. It makes me want to be of service to others and my environment. This continual developing awareness/connection between mind-body and spirit has been an essential in my walk on the planet.

Makara Adho Mukha Svanasana is one of my favorite asanas because it helps to tone just about my whole body and improves digestion. There is just so much to like about this pose. I've even been told that my arms look as good as Michelle Obama's!

The advice I would give to other curvy women who want to start yoga is be kind to yourself and just begin—practicing for 5-10 minutes a day is a great start. Leave judgment behind. Avoid taking yourself so seriously. There is always an opportunity to be spacious and BREATHE. Yoga is cheaper than drugs, psyche-therapy and it is totally yours. Mindfulness will never leave you.

Seneca's quote speaks to my truth. An individual's "truth" is his/her pillar of personal veracity, passion, personality and consciousness. This has been slightly bred out of most of us. Not trusting our own wisdom can be paralyzing because it manifests doubt and worry and prevents action.

I **love** my curves because they represent the divine feminine...strength, beauty, and connectivity.

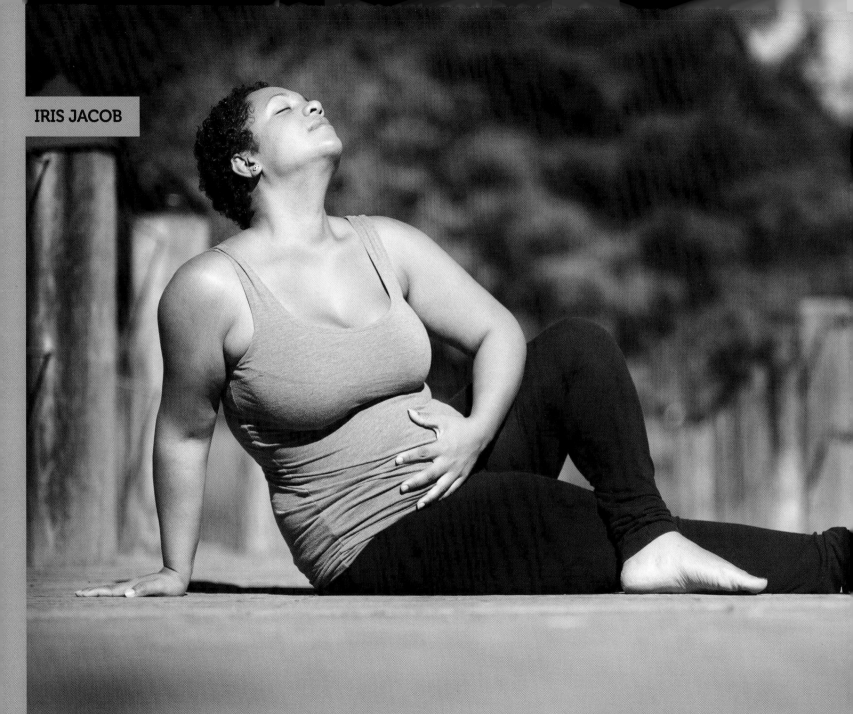

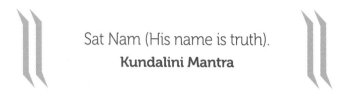

Sat Nam (His name is truth).
Kundalini Mantra

Marichyasana (MARICHI'S POSE)

Iris's Story...

I came to yoga two years ago when I was pregnant. I was hooked after my first class. I loved the way my body felt as I moved and stretched, feeling my baby moving and stretching inside of me. Standing in a strong warrior pose or as a goddess with my arms in prayer, belly protruding out, supported my belief in my power and abilities as a mother.

Bending myself into difficult, strength-building positions enabled me to enjoy an all-natural, homebirth. With yoga my body could do amazing things- like bring life into this world, and then heal itself.

I began taking Baby and Me Yoga classes after my daughter was born. In these classes, I was able to work on getting my body back in shape and bond with my daughter. I loved these classes so much I decided to teach them myself. Currently, I teach Baby and Me Yoga in Washington, DC.

My practice is about community and growth. When practicing with others, meditating and exchanging energy, I find that I feel beautiful, uplifted, and completely secure. In my own practice, and as I experiment with various types of yoga and poses, I am amazed at what my curvy, voluptuous, incredibly strong body can accomplish.

Marichyasana is one of my favorite poses, because it allows me to experiment with different mudras and ways to generate and express energy.

I **love** my curves because they are beautiful. Why wouldn't I love them?

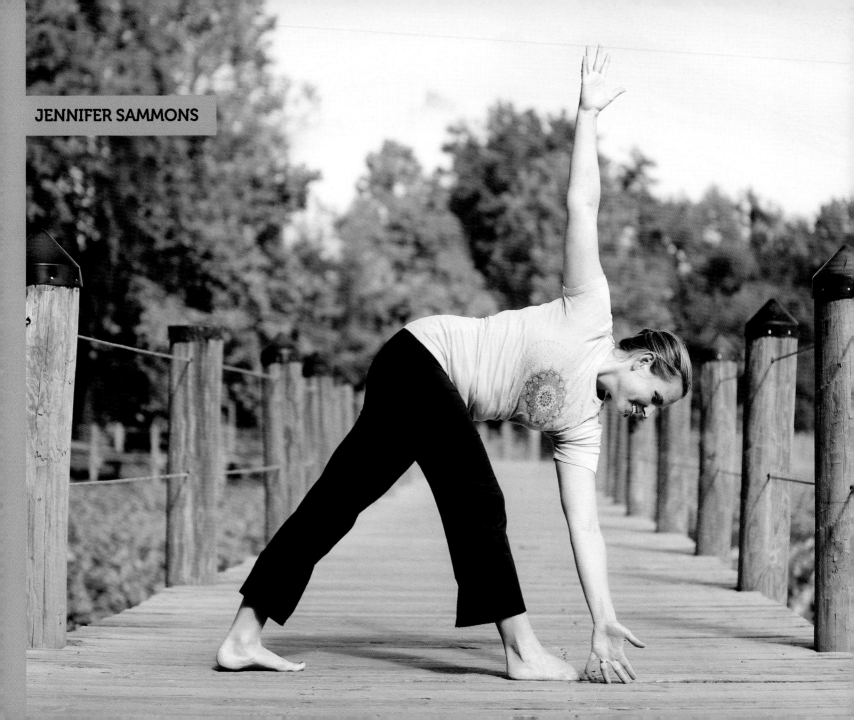

> Your present circumstances don't determine where you can go;
> they merely determine where you start.
> **Nido Qubein**

Parivrtta Trikonasana (REVOLVED TRIANGLE)

Jennifer's Story...

I started practicing 10 years ago after a bad breakup. I had moved and joined a new gym. I happened to take a yoga class, and the teacher was amazing. I went to every one of her classes, even a Monday night class that didn't end until 9 pm. (I am a morning person, so it is very unusual for me to choose to be at the gym past 7pm, especially when I had to leave for work by 5 am.) But it was worth it!

Yoga constantly reminds me that I need to be grateful for my body—for the strength that I have and what my body can achieve. I have also learned to be more forgiving toward my body.

Parivrtta Trikonasana is one of my favorite poses because it is challenging, and it makes me feel strong and powerful. It helps me stretch deeply. It allows me to release. I find myself saying "ah" each time that I come into it on my mat.

I chose the **Nido Qubein** quote because I often hear people say that they can't do yoga because they aren't flexible or don't have a sense of balance. That doesn't mean that you can't become more flexible or gain a firmer sense of balance. If we used our current circumstances as an excuse to not do something, we would never accomplish anything.

I **love** my curves because they remind me of what my body is able to produce— I love that I have even more curves since giving birth to my son.

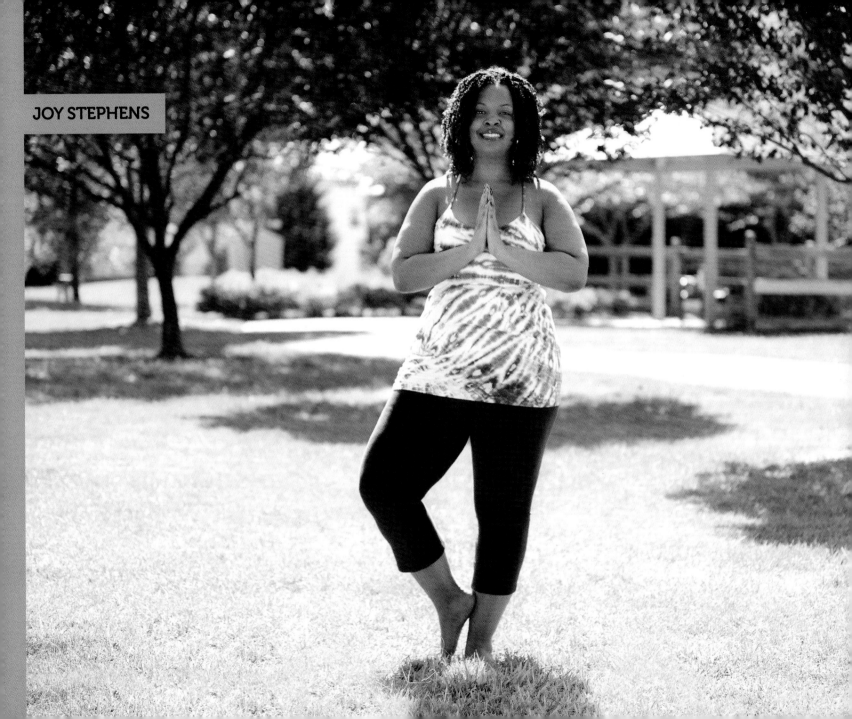

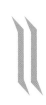

> *Start with yourself and healing will multiply.*
> **India.Irie**

Vrksasana (TREE POSE)

Joy's Story...

I've been practicing yoga for 10 years. Initially, I was inspired to start practicing for the physical benefits of yoga. Over the years, I began practicing mindfulness and found that yoga was essential to my overall well-being. Yoga feeds my body, mind, and spirit.

Yoga is truly for everybody. I love that my instructors encourage listening to our bodies, not comparing ourselves to others, and allowing for slight discomfort as we reach our edge. In my mind, these are great life principles. Yoga allows me to truly celebrate my body.

Vrksasana is one of my favorite poses because it evokes a sense of balance and stability. In this pose, I feel grounded and ready to take on new challenges. If I extend my arms, it reminds me of the possibilities that exist when I am standing on solid ground.

I chose the **India.Irie** quote because as a psychologist, I know self-care is essential to my well-being. In order to be of help to others, I have to be connected with my deepest self. Attending to my body, mind, and soul allows me to be present, mindful, and in tune with clients. It is also essential for my personal relationships.

I **love** my curves because they are divinely created.

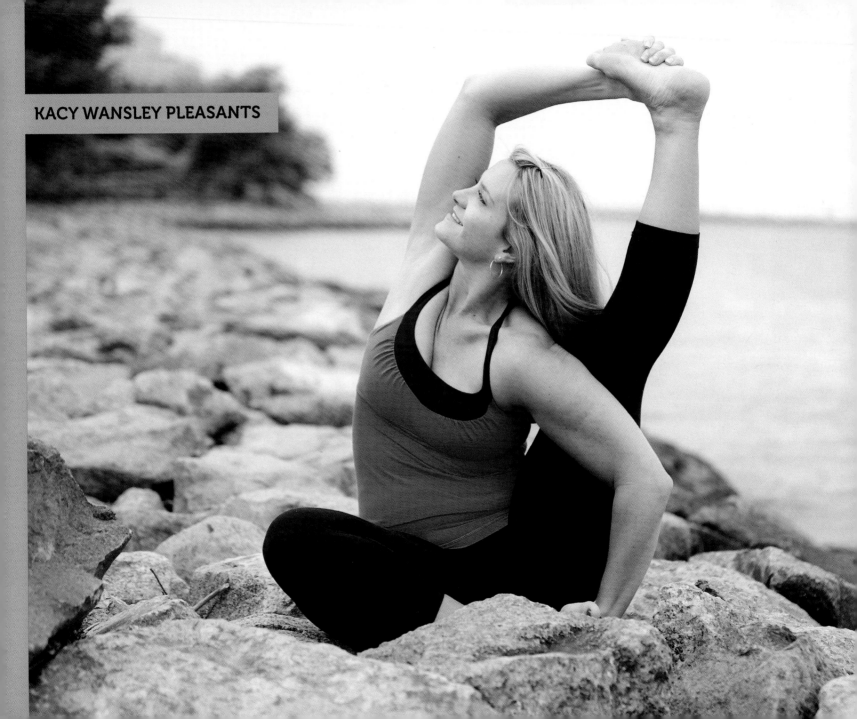

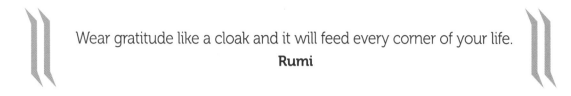

Wear gratitude like a cloak and it will feed every corner of your life.
Rumi

Parivrtta Surya Yantrasana (COMPASS POSE)

Kacy's Story...

I started practicing yoga five years ago, after the birth of my son. I was battling with depression. I turned to food and alcohol to stuff an empty hole and numb my pain. With the help of my supportive husband, I found help through therapy, and eventually yoga.

I love connecting to my breath on the mat and feeling powerful. Yoga helps me to realize that I am REAL. I'm a real woman with curves, stretch marks, and a beautiful soul. I am so grateful for what yoga has brought to my life.

Parivrtta Surya Yantrasana is one of my favorite asanas because it involves hip opening, side bending, and twisting. It makes me feel soft yet strong!

I chose the **Rumi** quote, because I really truly believe in gratitude and letting others know that you are thankful for them and thankful for what they do for you. Gratitude is what makes the world go round.

I **love** my curves because they belong to me. It took me a while to embrace them. I am now a yoga instructor. I remember feeling embarrassed in the sea of thin yoga teachers. I realize now that my curves make me real and approachable. My students relate to me. I am strong, flexible, and healthy.

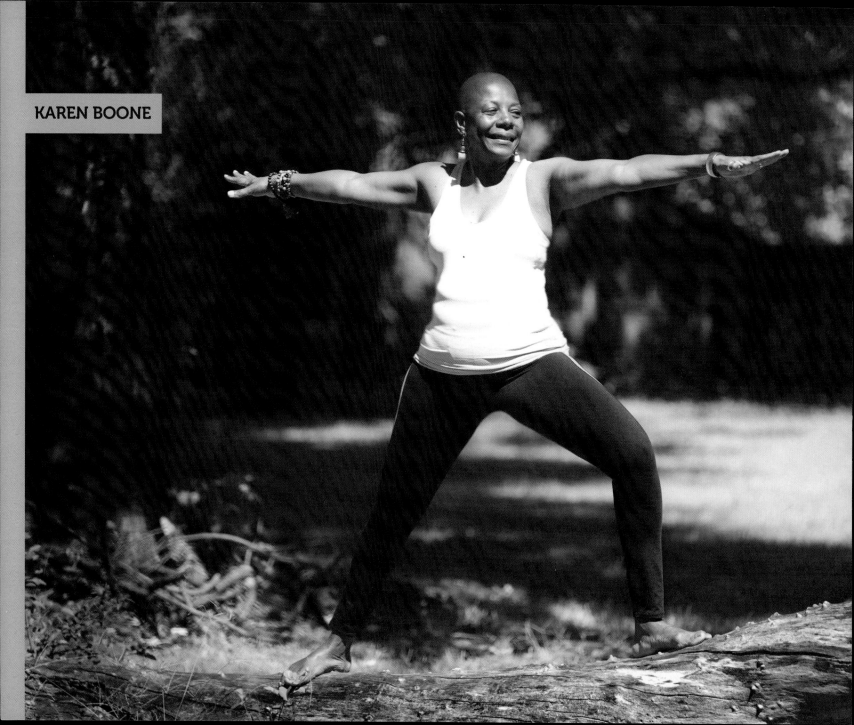

However long the night, the dawn will break.
African Proverb

Virabhadrasana II (WARRIOR II)

Karen's Story...

I've been practicing yoga for six years. A friend invited me to a yoga class, but I was apprehensive because I had preconceived ideas about yoga. I thought you had to look a certain way or be able to do certain things in order to practice. After much prodding, I finally went to a class. It was the most challenging thing I had done physically, but I felt good after the class was over. I wanted to continue to experience that same feeling and that's what started my journey.

Yoga helps me to connect with myself, the real me. It causes me to be mindful of my thoughts and feelings. Through yoga, I've learned that I am more than my physical body. Practicing yoga has helped me appreciate my body and be comfortable living in it.

Virabhadrasana II is one of my favorite poses as it simultaneously evokes feelings of power and peace. Whenever I am in this pose, I feel powerful and at the same time I feel balanced, centered, and in harmony with my true self.

I chose the quote because it gives me hope and lets me know that things will inevitably get better!

I **love** my curves because they make me uniquely who I am! And that's a good thing!

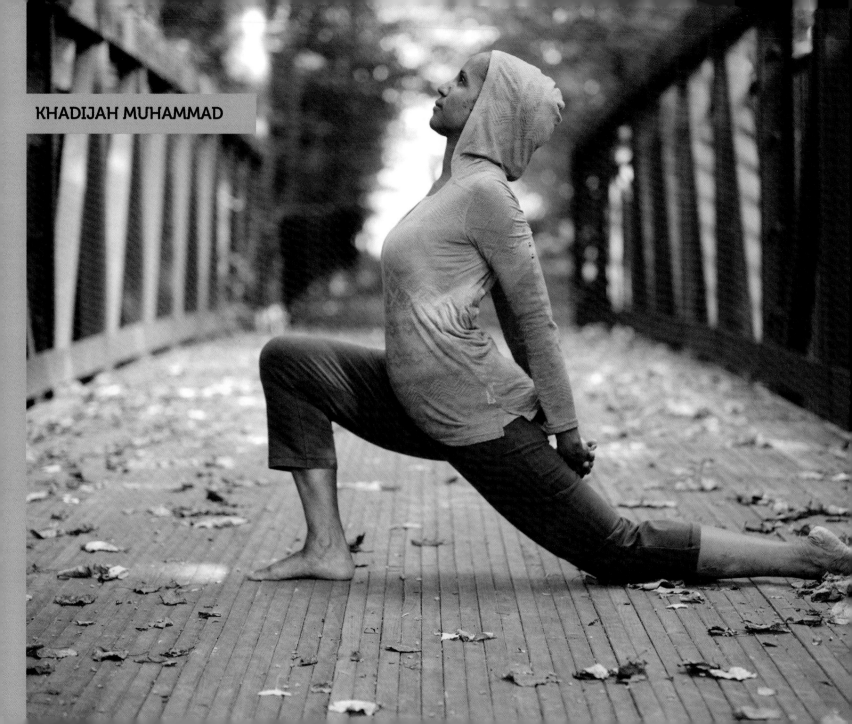

I am sick and tired of being sick and tired.
Fannie Lou Hamer

Anjaneyasana with Yoga Seal (LOW LUNGE)

Khadijah's Story...

I discovered yoga 11 years ago. I was seeking peace while grieving the death of my father. Yoga allows me to connect with and love my body better than any other physical activity. I enjoy all of the poses in the Sun Salutation sequence because my entire body is involved and engaged.

Anjaneyasana with the Yoga Mudra is one of my favorite asanas, because it allows my heart to feel open and unguarded. In the pose, my heart and gaze lift to receive as I send my love out to others: "Give and receive" is my mantra for wellness and balance.

The **Fannie Lou Hamer** quote speaks to me because when I made the decision to stop struggling with my body issues, family and personal problems, I gained the power to do better; to get better for me!

I **love** my curves because they show the true essence of my being.

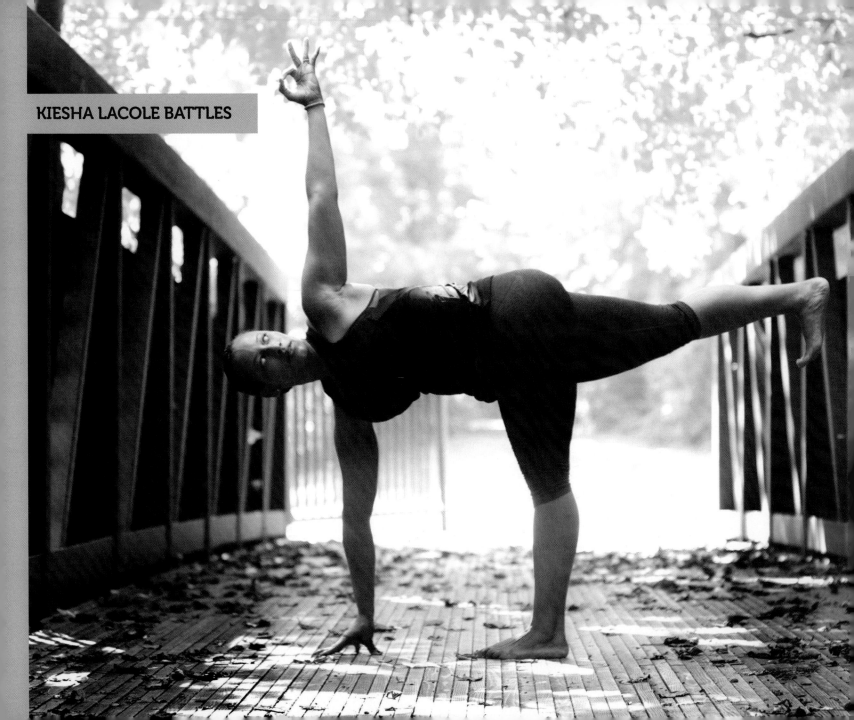

What each of us believes in is up to us,
but life is impossible without believing in something.
Kentetsu Takamori

Parivrtta Ardha Chandrasana (REVOLVED HALF MOON POSE)

Kiesha's Story...

I've been practicing yoga for 13 years. My inspiration to teach came in 2010, when my best friend asked me about my passions in life. That conversation was the spark that ignited my dedication to the practice of yoga and pushed me to pursue my goal of becoming an instructor.

When I was 15, my older brother died from HIV/AIDS. It was the worst experience of my life. But, it changed me in a positive way. His death shed light on the dark situations in my life. I learned to appreciate life and to live day-by-day, situation-by-situation.

My style of teaching is "YogaMe." When I think about what yoga is, it's truly an expression of the individual and where their body is at that moment. As I build and align my postures in my own practice, I can explore and choose what my body needs. Yoga presents so many options, allowing me to enjoy every posture.

Parivrtta Ardha Chandrasana is one of my favorite yoga poses because it requires strength to hold my thigh up in the sky, and send breath through all the straight lines of my limbs and twist my torso open. It amazes me that in the midst of all of that, my mind finds the ease required to maintain balance in the pose. My fears are released as I gaze high forgetting what's below.

I **love** my curves because they represent who I am. I come from a long line of curvy women: my mother, my grandmother, and my cousin. I love me, so of course I love my firm, sagging, turning, and hanging curves.

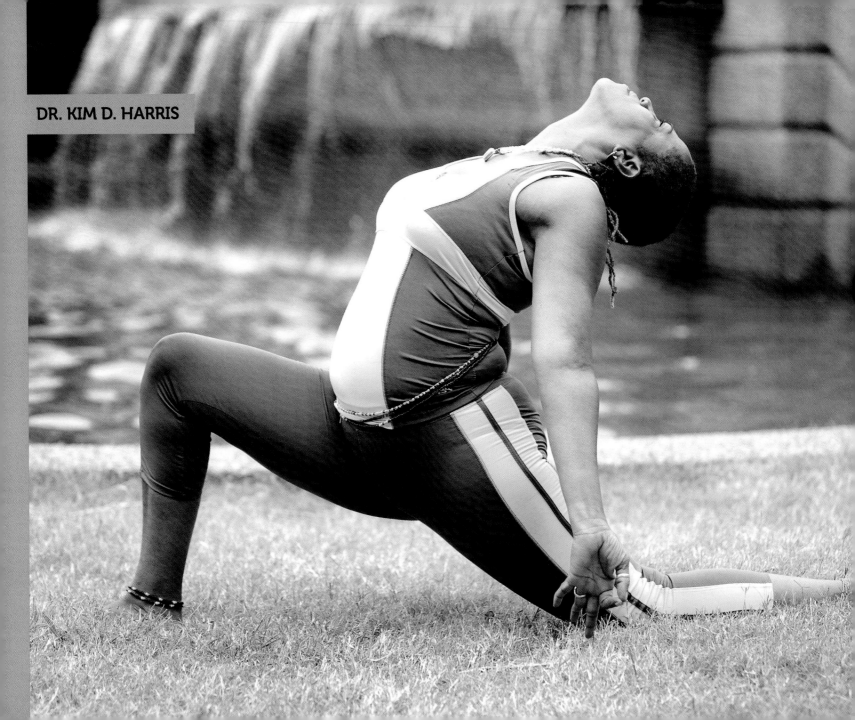

DR. KIM D. HARRIS

Anjaneyasana with Yoga Hasta Mudra
(LOW LUNGE WITH YOGA HAND GESTURE)

Kim's Story...

I have been practicing yoga for three years. I was inspired to practice yoga during my stint with breast cancer. As a healing modality, the practice of yoga gave me an opportunity to reconnect to myself with an attitude of gratitude. As I move, stretch, and breathe, I celebrate the presence of my body. As I move, stretch, and breathe, I depict love for my body maintaining a laser focus of balance being ready and steady to move, stretch, and breathe.

I am totally immersed with the rule of four-breathing as means to maintain balance while engaged with this **Anjaneyasana** variation. This pose incites energy sensations throughout my mind, body, and soul as my hips open and my chest, lungs, and shoulders expand. I always feel empowered with a sense of deep self-reflection about how good it is to be divinely alive.

This **Bhagvad Gita** quote is symbolic of my journey as a Basu (a title given when completing a certification via the Tjef Neteru Sema Paut, a system of Kemetic Yoga). The journey presented many challenges for me as a breast cancer survivor as my range of motion was limited due to my mastectomy. But I kept practicing, and consistency led to a deeper connection between me, my practice, and the mat.

I **love** my curves because they authentically define the entire me.

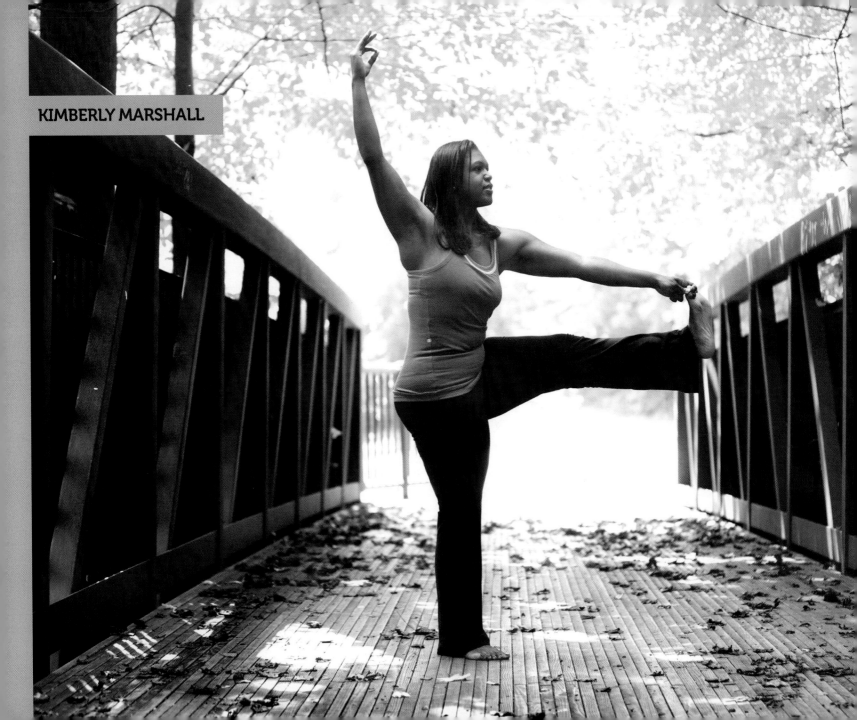

KIMBERLY MARSHALL

> Success is where preparation and opportunity meet!
> **Bobby Unser**

Eka Pada Hasta Padangusthasana (HAND TO BIG TOE POSE)

Kimberly's Story...

I've been practicing yoga for about five years. I discovered yoga while looking for a way to quiet my mind and focus. Yoga helps to get me to a great place of mental and spiritual clarity. Yoga also makes me feel strong and graceful. It helps reinforce my abilities and makes me push myself beyond what I think I am capable of and what others might expect.

Eka Pada Hasta Padangusthasana is one of my favorite poses because it exemplifies the strength and flexibility that I have come to discover through my practice.

The **Bobby Unser** quote reminds me to always work on progressing and presenting my best self, so I can take advantage of any opportunity whenever it presents itself.

I **love** my curves because they are what make me a woman.

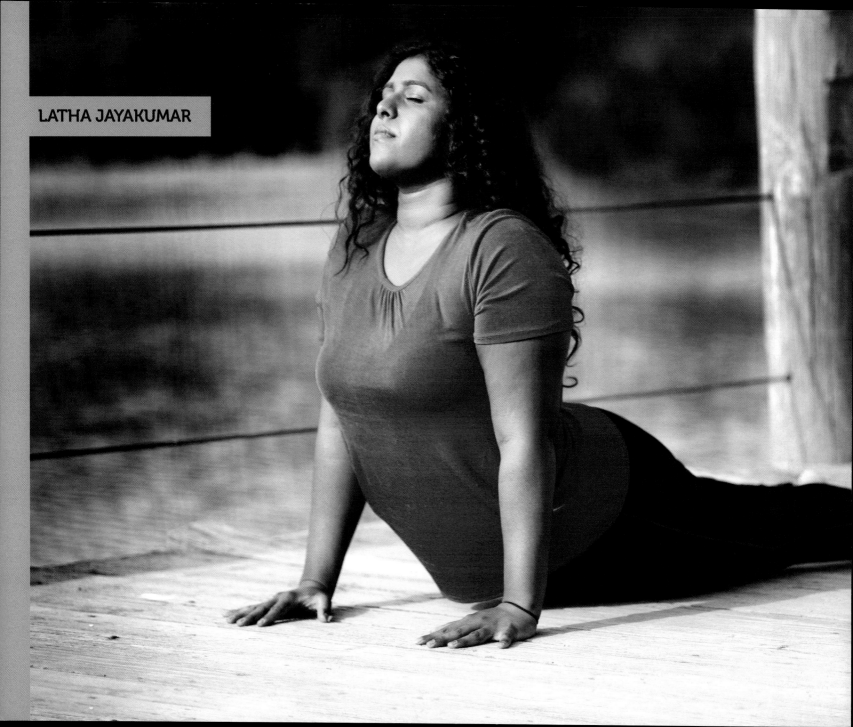

If you can believe it, you can achieve it!
Unknown

Urdhva Mukha Svanasana (UPWARD FACING DOG POSE)

Latha's Story...

My grandmother taught me little pieces of yoga here and there all my life. I only became serious about it in the last two years, when I decided to get my teaching certification. I realized my body was aging faster than I wanted it to. I started to notice how inflexible I was becoming and I didn't want that to happen. Yoga has helped me counteract the effects of aging, due to a job that requires me to sit at the computer most of the day.

Yoga helps keep my body and mind active. I love the shape of my body with all its curves, and I love how yoga helps me stay limber and keeps my curves beautiful. I use my practice to realign my mind. All day I am bombarded with images of rail thin models. I take time in my practice to love my body for the way it is.

Urdhva Mukha Svanasana is one of my favorite poses because I feel strong when I do it. Also as an asthma sufferer from a very young age, I enjoy how the pose opens up my accessory muscles of breathing in my chest. It is a therapeutic pose that really give me a good stretch.

I chose that quote because it is something I live by every day. I believe that we create the events and path our lives take and that anything is truly possible. We are unlimited.

I **love** my curves because they are a part of me. They are beautiful and make me unique.

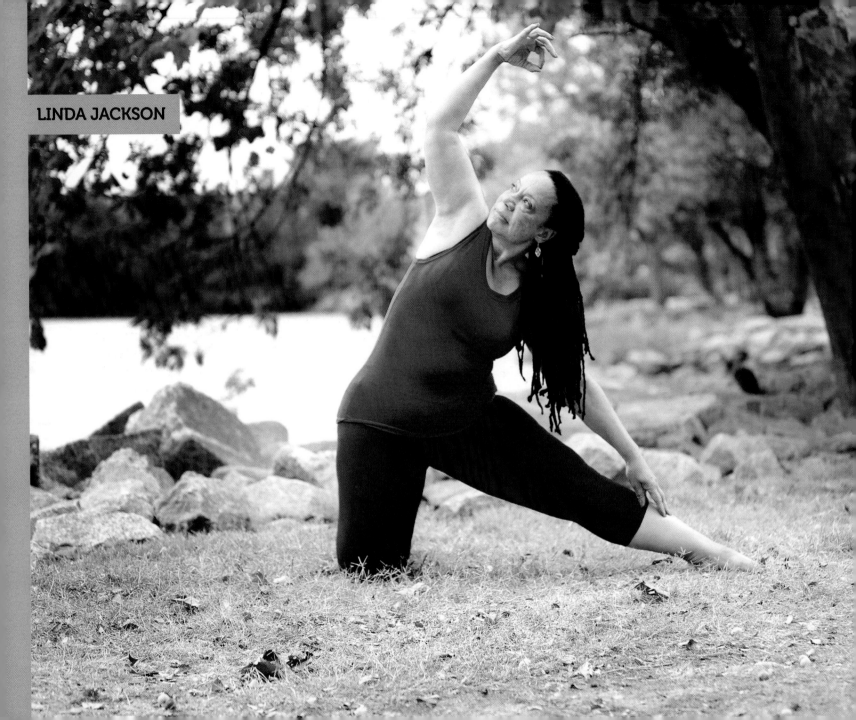

LINDA JACKSON

Parighasana (GATE POSE)

Linda's Story...

I came to yoga two years ago in an effort to heal a knee problem. Initially, my doctor recommended physical therapy or arthroscopic surgery to treat my knee. However, I wanted a treatment that I could take responsibility for, rather than one that was done to me. So, I changed doctors. My new orthopedic surgeon also recommended physical therapy. Surprisingly, the physical therapist helped me understand how yoga was a lifestyle choice that would help improve my health. At the end of my last PT session, he said, "No one will ever love you more than you love yourself." I reflect on his wise words nearly every day.

Yoga also helped me bond with my father during our final vacation together last summer. We did chair yoga together. My dad practiced every asana to the best of his ability. He understood yoga, and he understood me. He died a few months later, but the time we spent together helped me to accept his passing.

This quote by **Satchidananda** speaks to my soul. I am, by nature, a joyous person and this quote helps me to remember to live a life of joy.

Parighasana is one of my favorite poses because it represents the joy of the journey. When I'm in the pose, I can see the destination, reach toward it, release everything that has held me back, and flow toward the destination. Parighasana represents my yoga journey. I am continuing my journey to the destination, even as the destination constantly changes.

I **love** my curves because my body is and will always be the vessel of my soul, no matter what shape or size.

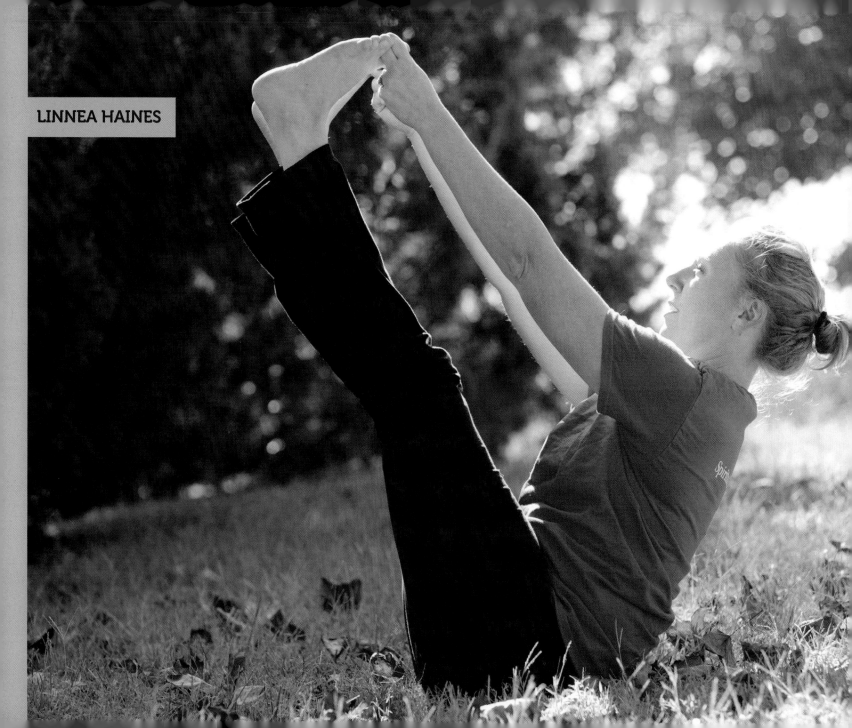

LINNEA HAINES

Navasana (BOAT POSE)

Linnea's Story...

I've been practicing yoga for over 23 years. I was drawn to yoga because of how it connects and strengthens the mind and body. For me, yoga is about accepting and loving yourself for who you are and where you are today; while you work toward a higher goal and toward achieving greater enlightenment. It's about self-actualization.

Navasana is one of my favorite yoga poses because it helps with stabilization and core and supports so many other poses. I feel like having a stabilized core keeps me grounded in all areas of my life. It prevents me from overreacting or taking life too seriously. It enables me to keep things in perspective, and to give my energy to those things that are the most important, while letting inconsequential things go.

Mother Theresa's quote speaks to me because even when we think we have nothing left to give and life is more challenging than we can handle, there is always love that can lift us, and we are each other's guiding lights and saving graces. The Lord works through us to show His love to His children.

I **love** my curves because my they are a visual celebration of my being a woman.

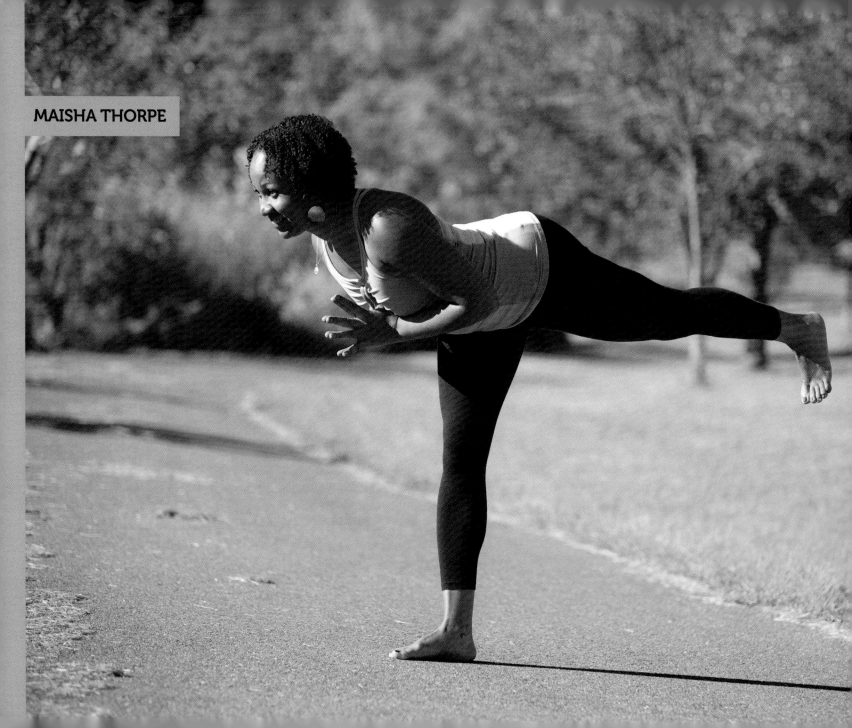

MAISHA THORPE

BE Bold. BE Real. BE Full. BE Present.
Personal Mantra

Virabhadrasana III (WARRIOR III)

Maisha's Story...

I started practicing yoga in 2005, during my first pregnancy, and continued recreationally off and on post-delivery. I also began running 5Ks and even completed a half marathon in 2007. Yoga was a good cross training option for me.

I started taking my practice deeper in 2012, when I began to understand the benefits of yoga and meditation for relieving stress. Seeking more formal instruction and a community of like minds led me to take classes at Spiritual Essence Yoga with Dana. The study of yoga opened me up to a lifestyle change that allows me to be intentional about every day and attentive to my mind, body, and spirit.

Virabhadrasana III is one of my favorite poses, because it embodies my need to embrace balance in my life. I especially like that all of the muscles are engaged in the pose. It helps me quiet my mind and focus while building core strength. Also known as Warrior 3, this powerful standing asana gives me a feeling of strength and endurance.

My **personal mantra** inspires me daily: BE Bold. BE Real. BE Full. BE Present. "Be Bold," reminds me to initiate always. "Be Real," is to speak my truth. "Be Full," is to be safe and comfortable within myself. Lastly, "Be Present," reminds me to enjoy living in the moment. My mantra is my daily compass and my barometer for inner peace.

I **love** my curves because they represent my life's journey.

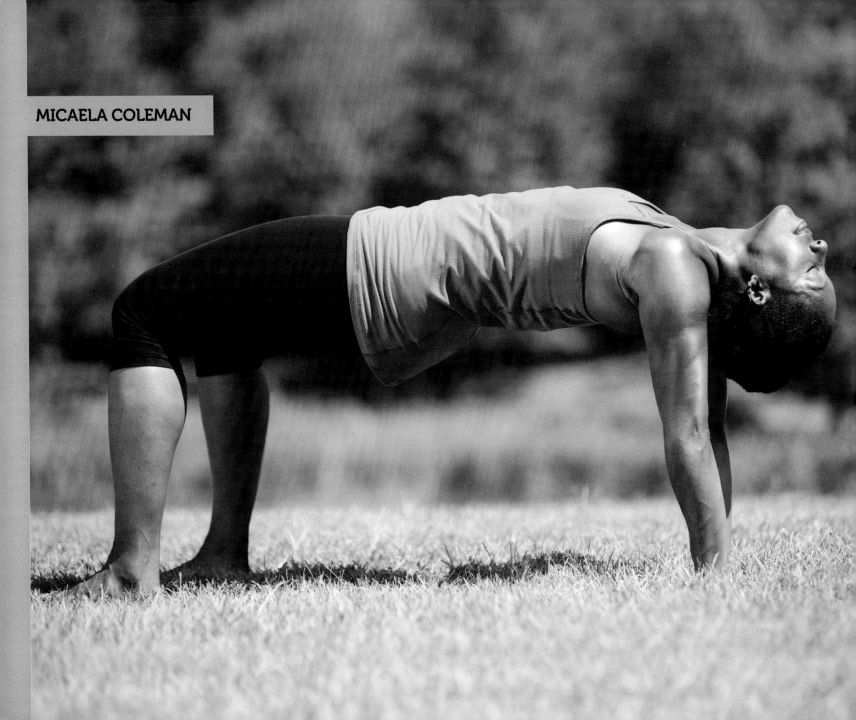

MICAELA COLEMAN

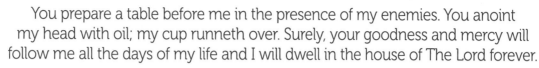

You prepare a table before me in the presence of my enemies. You anoint my head with oil; my cup runneth over. Surely, your goodness and mercy will follow me all the days of my life and I will dwell in the house of The Lord forever.

Psalm 23:5-6

Ardha Purvottanasana (HALF UPWARD PLANK POSE)

Micaela's Story...

I have been faithfully practicing yoga for the past three years. In 2010, an orthopedic physician instructed me to adopt new lifestyle habits as a means of addressing post-accident injuries to my cervical spine. He recommended lengthening and strengthening my muscles through yoga or Pilates, I chose yoga.

Through yoga, I found peace, open-mindedness, and the freedom to explore my inner self with acceptance of my limitations. Little did I know that the meditative aspects of Kundalini, Reiki, and pranayama would lead me to expand my journey into a 200-hour yoga teacher training program. I am now sharing yoga at Evolutions Yoga in Greenwood, IN.

Ardha Purvottanasana is one of my favorite asanas, because it stretches my shoulders, chest, and strengthens my wrists. It is a challenge for me to find good alignment in this pose, but when I do it serves as proof that I am overcoming a neck injury that has been part of my new normal for the past four years. As with other unexpected occurrences in life, to fully experience Ardha Purvottanasana, I must modify in order to fully realize my potential. To me, this asana invokes determination.

The **Psalm** reminds me that God will provide in spite of the naysayers and the dark gloom that looms at times. He'll give the enemy a reason to get mad just as soon as they see how He's chosen to bless you.

I **love** my curves because of their distinct shape and for how they have become more defined over the years.

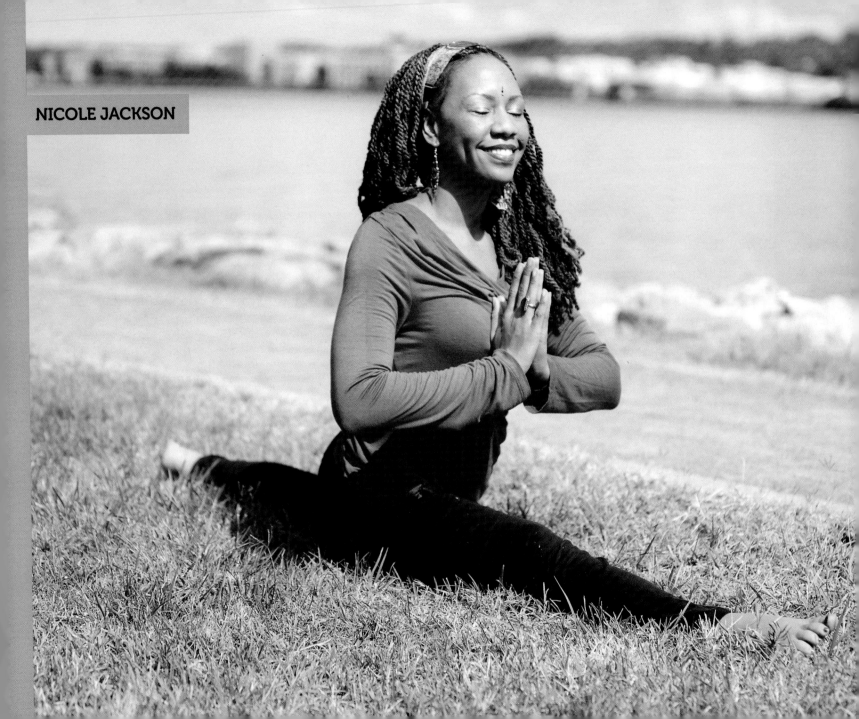

> Everything is always in divine and perfect order.
>
> **Unknown**

Hanumanasana (MONKEY POSE/SPLIT)

Nicole's Story...

I rediscovered yoga in 2007, and I have been practicing for over five years. I say "rediscovered" because I feel yoga has been with me over many incarnations. I was inspired to start practicing yoga this time around by my spirit guides in my quest for aligning with my spiritual purpose. I was led to my first yoga book, "Chakra Yoga," written by Alan Finger, which at the time was so intriguing to me because I had just recently discovered the world of Reiki, chakras, and energy healing. Yoga came to me in a transitional period, a time when I needed it the most. Through yoga, I was given a spiritual practice, a method that allowed me to further my journey of self-healing and self-discovery. It helped me to connect with my inner divinity and to attain more balance in my life. I was able to transform my body and mind.

Yoga helps me to love myself as I am. Through connecting with the divine essence within, I am reminded that I am perfect as I am. Through yoga, I can celebrate the feminine energy that my curves represent. I celebrate all women, for we are all one.

Hanumanasana is a powerful hip opener, thigh and hamstring stretch. For me, the pose represents the significance of surrendering and letting go. It reminds me to release the things, thoughts, and emotions that do not serve me, such as tension in my body. I appreciate this pose because it facilitates greater strength, openness, and lightness within my lower body and heart center.

The quote inspires me because it's the truth! We must remind ourselves of this truth even when going through hard times. There is always a divine plan at work. So be encouraged and know that in the end, it was always for your greater good, and of the greater good of all.

I **love** my curves because they are part of me, and well, simply put... I love all of me!

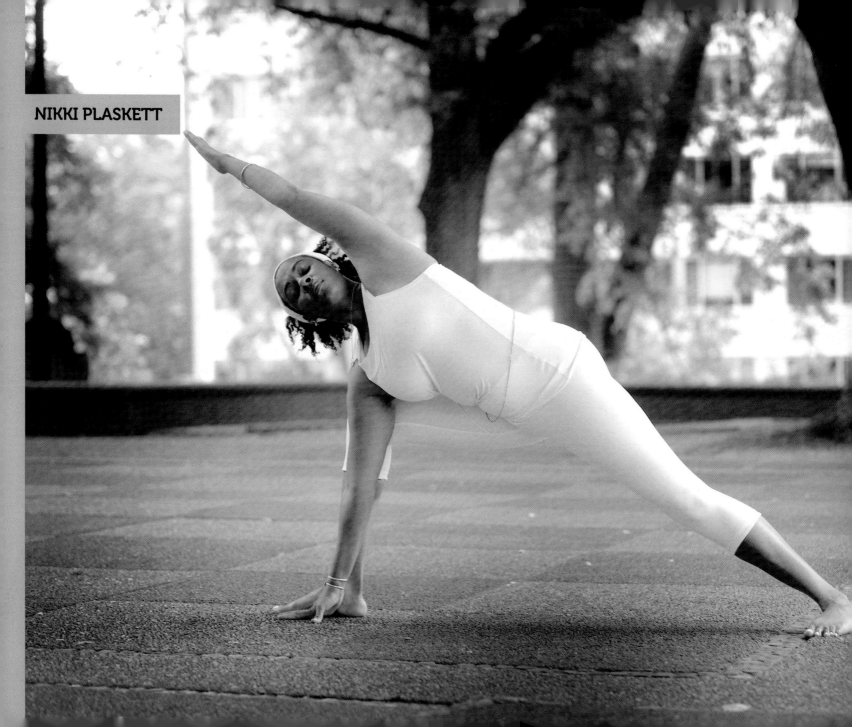

NIKKI PLASKETT

Uttitha Parsvakonasana (EXTENDED SIDE ANGLE POSE)

Nikki's Story...

I've been practicing yoga on and off since childhood and consistently for the past 14 years. Yoga offers me a blank slate to start over and over again with each breath. It keeps me intimately connected to the nooks and crannies that go unnoticed in our culture. I have to confront every fold and feel my girth to assume some postures. Some days practice can be quite funky, both emotionally and olfactory, and I realize that it's time to cleanse and clear out the clutter. Whiles other days my flow is light, airy, and long, allowing space, extension and projection arrive pleasantly with such grace.

Parsvakonasana is an expansive pose, and I love the energy it releases. It encourages me to open my treasure chest (the heart and groin) and expose them to the universe. It awakens my heart and creative centers and simultaneously grounds me back to the earth as I root and center my weight over both feet. It raises me to the heavens as I rotate my torso and reach out through my fingertips. Stamina and endurance abounds with each breath I take as my ribs and side body open. Parsvakonasana engages my whole body. It provides the opportunity to focus the macro into micro: I can lose myself fine tuning through the sweat of this asana, or I can gaze up and meditate in action.

Yogiji's quote inspires me because it reminds me to take time and take care of myself, so I can take care of others. It reminds me to allow myself the same compassion, forgiveness, and acceptance I would to a friend. Essentially, fighting with someone else requires you to hurt and fight with yourself.

I **love** my curves because they are softer than corners, divinely feminine, and fluid. When I visualize abstractions of water and air I see curves, ocean waves and jet streams are curvy. Life is curvy.

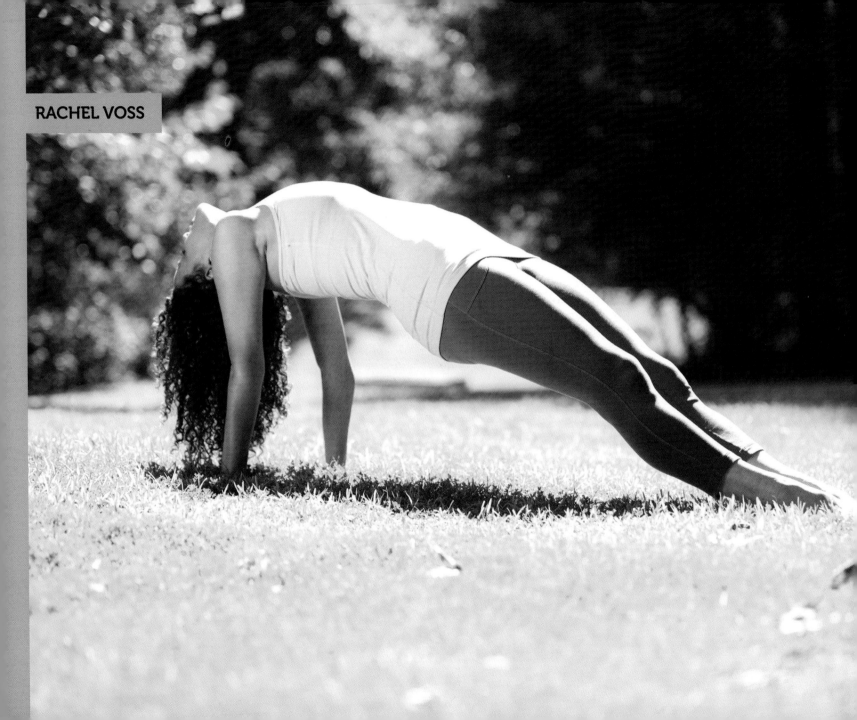

RACHEL VOSS

> There is no need of competition with anybody.
> You are yourself and as you are, you are perfectly good. Accept yourself.
>
> **Osho**

Purvottanasana (INCLINED PLANK POSE)

Rachel's Story...

Yoga has always been in my life, but I've been practicing consistently since 2012. I have many yoga inspirations in my life; mainly my stepmother, who I grew up watching practice yoga. I've always wanted to practice it to achieve the level of Zen that my stepmother has achieved. In June 2012, my practice was kicked into full gear as a result of a car accident. I started practicing to help heal my physical body, which led to the journey of spiritual and emotional healing.

The more I continue to see my body do things I never thought it could do, and I mean even just touching my toes, the more I have developed an appreciation for the body I was given. In learning to love myself more, I have learned to fully embrace my wonderful curves. Yoga has been my place of peace, stability, strength and a renewed sense of self.

Purvottanasana is one of my favorite poses, because it is one of those poses that may look easy, but is challenging to do in its full expression. In this pose, I am able to ground myself using the strength of my whole body. I feel this asana in every area of my body. It makes my body feel powerful and connected.

Yoga has taught me the importance of looking within for healing, strength, and peace. This quote seems to speak to that truth. Our individual self is all we can control. I always refer to this quote when I need a reminder of my own personal greatness. It also speaks to my journey on the mat. In yoga, we are taught not to compare our journey with anyone else's, as well as not to compete with others or with ourselves. We are reminded in yoga to accept our bodies and ourselves exactly as we are.

I **love** my curves because of how womanly they make me feel, and because they are God's special gift designed just for my body.

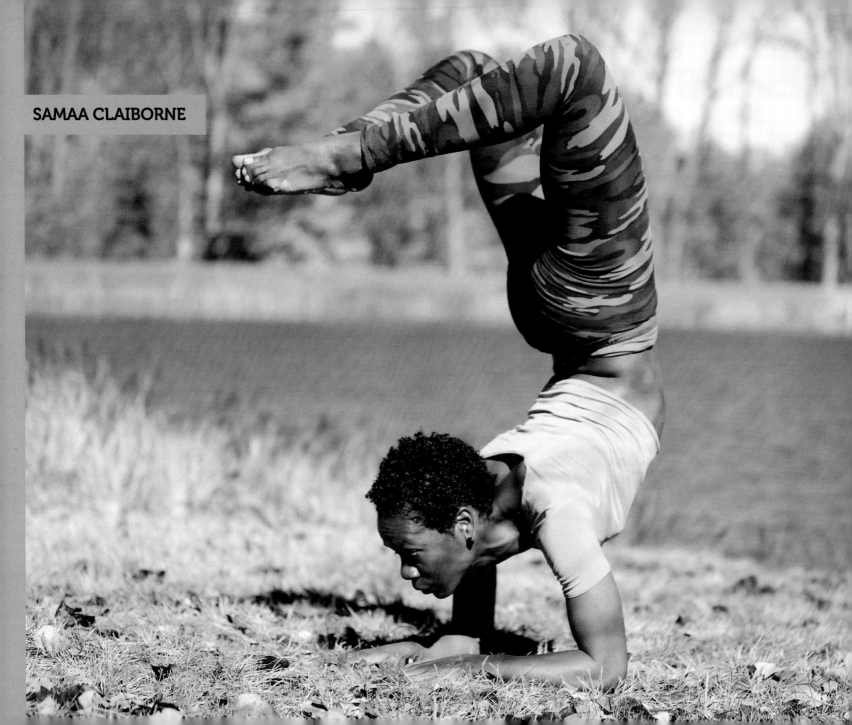

SAMAA CLAIBORNE

I could die here. Make my limbs like a tree. Place each thought in a leaf.
Fix my posture so that my grandchildren's backs are straight.

HawaH

Vrischikasana (SCORPION POSE)

Samaa's Story...

I've been practicing yoga for eight years. I was inspired to start practicing by an exceptionally gorgeous yogi who wanted to practice with me! I am grateful for the discipline that I've achieved as a result of my practice. When I can stand on the palms of my hands with my toes pointing straight towards the ceiling, trust me, it's cause for celebration! It takes cultivating discipline to achieve that level of strength and balance. I don't doubt that the discipline becomes engrained inside my veins and encourages confidence in my body and its capabilities. There's definitely a love affair happening between my body and yoga.

Vrischikasana is one of my favorite asanas because it requires me to be in a space of single-pointed focus. Bending back in the pose simultaneously opens and exposes the heart, which allows vulnerability to fully occupy the self. Personally, there's a shedding that occurs when I'm in this pose. With mindfulness, I'm actively releasing unwanted energy through the crown of the head and creating more space in the breathing centers of my body.

The **HawaH** quote connects me to the author so deeply, especially since he's my best friend, former lover, and the one that introduced me to yoga. But more than that, each time I read this, it immediately connects me to the things that nourish me the most –the breath, yoga, trees, my core, my child, the GREAT MOTHER EARTH, stability, and love. It also reminds me to lengthen through my spine!

I **love** my curves because I want them to love me as I age with grace.

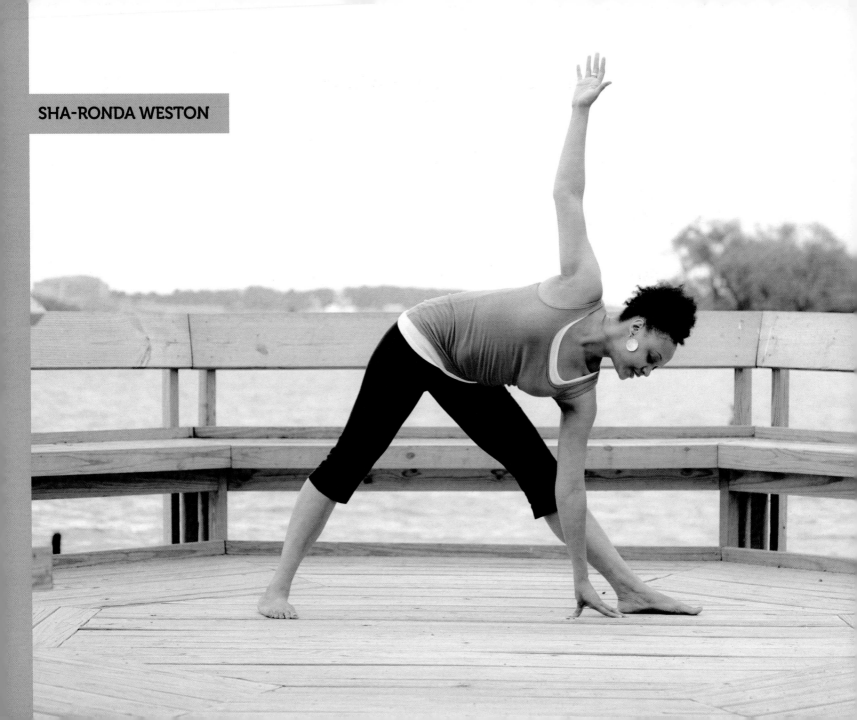

It's not what you GO through in life; it's what you GROW through in life.

Unknown

Trikonasana (TRIANGLE POSE)

Sha-Ronda's Story...

Yoga has been a part of my life for nine years. I was inspired to practice by watching my best friend, who experienced so many benefits through yoga. Yoga allows me to relax and accept myself as I am. Yoga is very calming. It allows me to spend time with myself and to commune with God. I am able to breathe in positive energy and release negativity. I feel powerful and strong in mind, body, and spirit after each practice.

My advice to other curvy women who are interested in yoga is, don't look at the person on the magazine or even on the mat next to you because they are not YOU. Yoga is not about a body type or age; it's about getting in touch with your inner you. Focus on you and learn to enjoy who YOU really are. In turn, you just might find the inner peace and love you are searching for.

Trikonasana is one of my favorite poses, because it makes me feel strong and balanced. I have to cast all my cares away and truly focus when getting into and more importantly, staying in this pose. The pose tones my arms and legs, engages my core, and stretches my whole body. It makes me feel open and free both physically and mentally. It is a go-to pose for whenever I have had a stressful day.

The quote I chose really speaks to me. We all face challenges in our daily lives, but our response to these experiences truly shapes who we are and guides us on this journey called life.

I **love** my curves because they are unique to me.

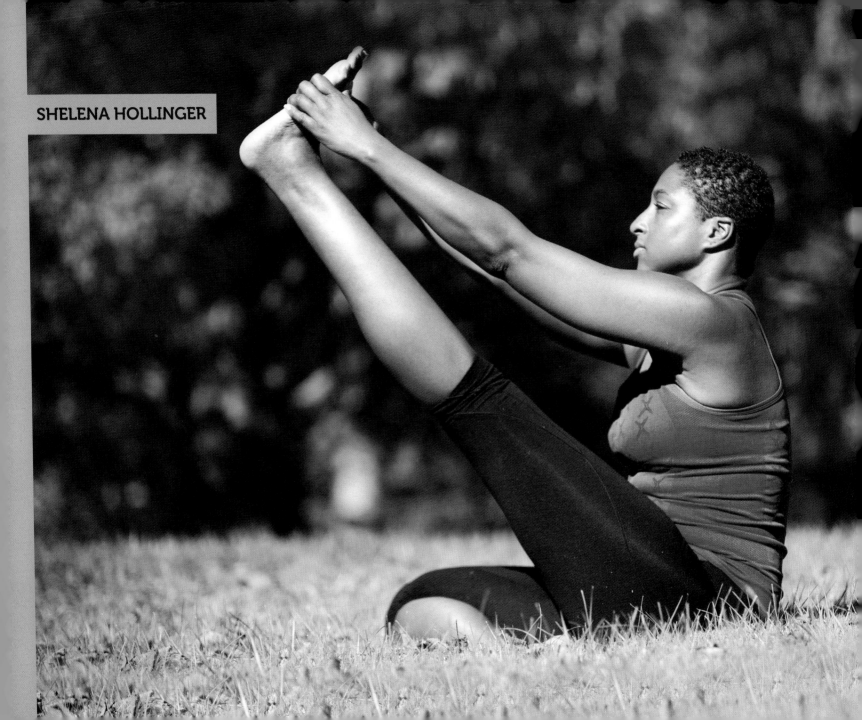

SHELENA HOLLINGER

> Being happy doesn't mean that everything is perfect.
> It means you've decided to look beyond the imperfections.
>
> **Unknown**

Krounchasana (HERON POSE)

Shelena's Story...

I've been practicing yoga for 10 years. I worked with Dana in the corporate world. We had a lot in common, we were both busy mommies. I was inspired by Dana's desire to improve her quality of life, and I wanted to help her achieve her dreams and desires. She introduced me to a lifestyle that I knew very little about.

Yoga helps me celebrate and love my curves because it reminds me that my body can still move, bend, and be strong. More importantly, I learned that there's room for growth: I can move more, bend more, and become an even stronger woman.

Krounchasana is one of my favorite poses because I like challenges. I've had three knee surgeries and two shoulder surgeries. I thought I would NEVER be able to practice yoga. I have overcome many hurdles in my recovery. Dana has given me guidance and suggestions over the years. Krounchasana reminds me that I am an overcomer. Through yoga I've learned patience and diligence. Every day I practice, I find I can do a little bit more than the day before.

The quote speaks to me because although things may not be perfect, you can always choose to love the moment you're in, regardless of what it brings you.

I **love** my curves because they validate me. I have become the woman I desired to be from childhood.

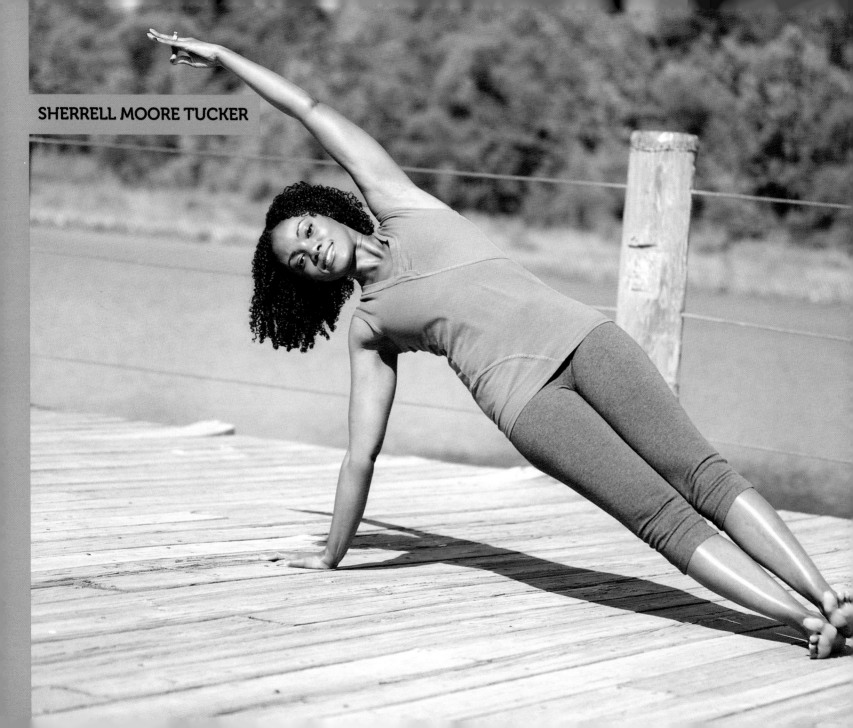

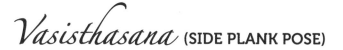

> Freedom is not worth having if it does not include the freedom to make mistakes.
>
> **M. K. Gandhi**

Vasisthasana (SIDE PLANK POSE)

Sherrell's Story...

I've been practicing yoga for approximately five years. After numerous failed attempts at physical therapy to alleviate arthritis pain in my lower back, the therapist recommended yoga. Yoga helps me to celebrate my curves through the common use of modifications that work with and not against my body.

Vasisthasana is one of my favorite yoga poses because I feel strength in it. I have some knee and lower back challenges. This poses reminds me that I am strong, and that I am progressing. Balancing on one hand and the side of one foot is something that I've never done before, so when I need that extra "boost" I embrace Vasisthasana and it embraces me.

If you are curvy and would like to start yoga, I say give it a shot! Although yoga is for everybody, not every studio or instructor is for everybody. Do your research and find an instructor and studio space where you feel comfortable and supported.

I am connected to the quote by **Gandhi** because freedom allows for success and failures, both of which are needed to build character.

I **love** my curves because my curves are unique to me and to my personality.

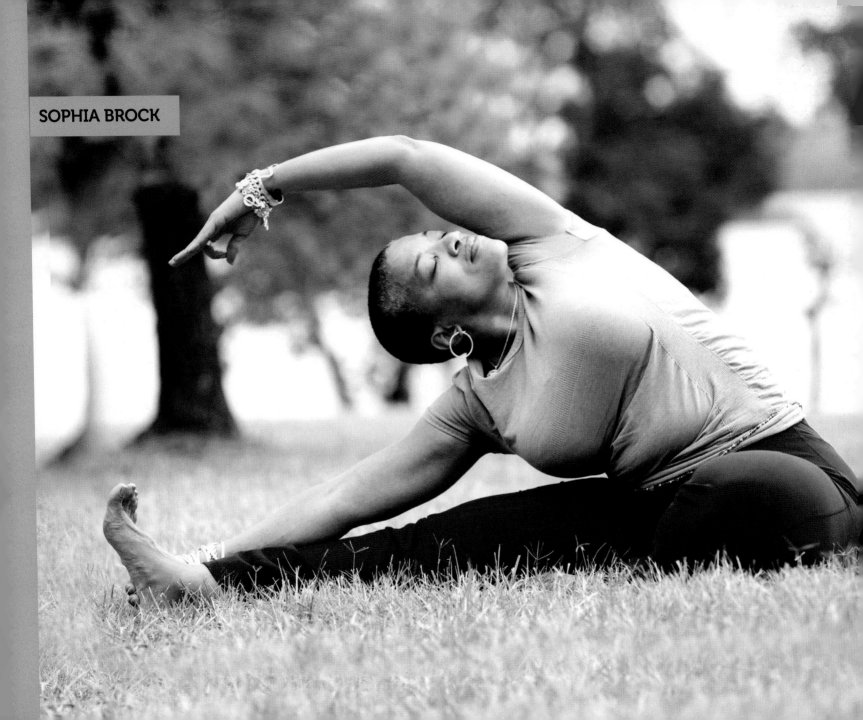

SOPHIA BROCK

If you cant see GOD in All you cant see GOD at all
Yogi Bhajan

Janu Sirsasana (HEAD TO KNEE POSE)

Sophia's Story...

I've been practicing yoga since 2003. I started out of curiosity, and the way I felt afterward inspired me to return. Yoga is honest. If you listen it will reveal what you need more or less of. Yoga helps me continuously embrace my ever changing body. It allows me to celebrate and love all that my body can, and cannot do.

Janu Sirsasana encourages me to surrender and breathe (a great recipe for living well). It also allows me to go "inside," myself. After a good warm up, I can move into Janu Sirsasana, close my eyes, and hang out in the pose with ease.

Yogi Bhajan's quote speaks to me because I know once you can see God in all, you have truly arrived (or returned).

I **love** my curves because they are mine—I don't deny them, and I don't hide them. My curves embolden me.

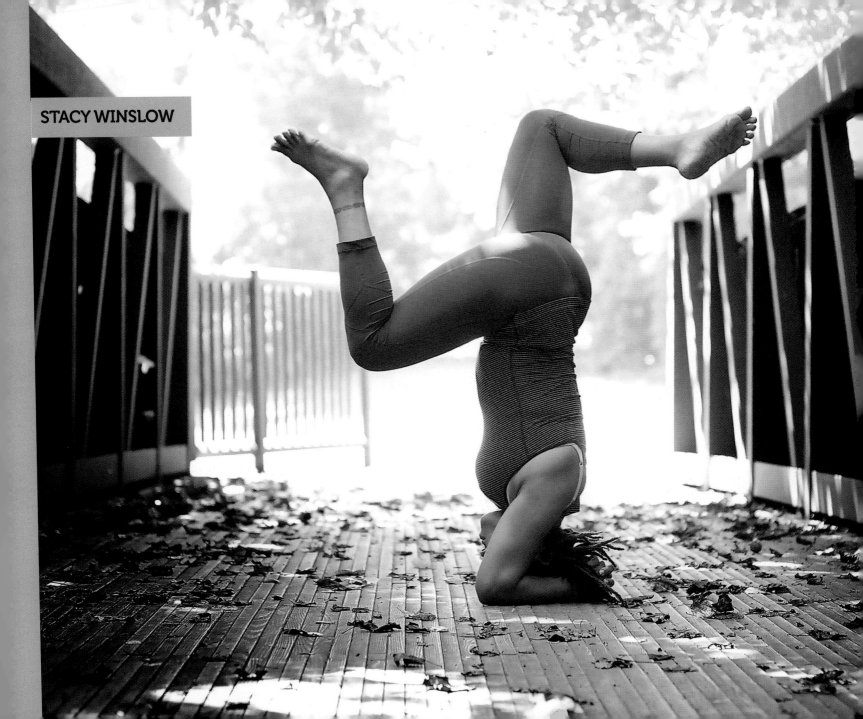

STACY WINSLOW

> To whom much is given, much is required.
> **Luke 12:48**

Sirsasana (HEADSTAND)

Stacy's Story...

I've been practicing yoga for 10 years. I was a young mother at the beginning of my fitness journey, and my local gym offered a yoga class. I took the class, and it was an awful experience. The teacher had no idea how to make asana accessible to a curvy body. So, I began a home practice until I found a yoga studio that taught me how to use props. But most importantly, the studio introduced me to the philosophy of yoga and eventually yoga teacher training.

Yoga helps me love and celebrate my body. It joins my mind and body in the present moment. Yoga has opened me up to experiencing the full gamut of human emotion without getting lost in it. I can take in joy, love, sorrow, pain, and forgiveness, and remain present. Practicing the balance between ease and effort has caused me to feel like a true force of grace.

Sirsasana is one of my favorite poses because it makes me feel grounded. When I first tried Sirsasana, I tried it against a wall because I was afraid of falling. But I quickly learned that I had the physical ability to support my own weight. When I moved away from the wall, I'll be honest, I did fall a time or two. Although falling was frightening, I fell safely into a lovely backbend. Falling is another wonderful part of my yogic journey. It teaches me that I can face a scary situation and safely face it again! And again! That is empowering. For me, Sirsasana embodies my inner victory that was built upon a strong foundation.

The **Bible verse** speaks to me because most people, particularly in the U.S., live abundant lives. Unfortunately most people also take their abundance for granted. An attitude of gratitude is the backbone of a life well lived. Giving back is a way of life for me and it is how my parents raised me.

I **love** my curves because they make me feel powerful.

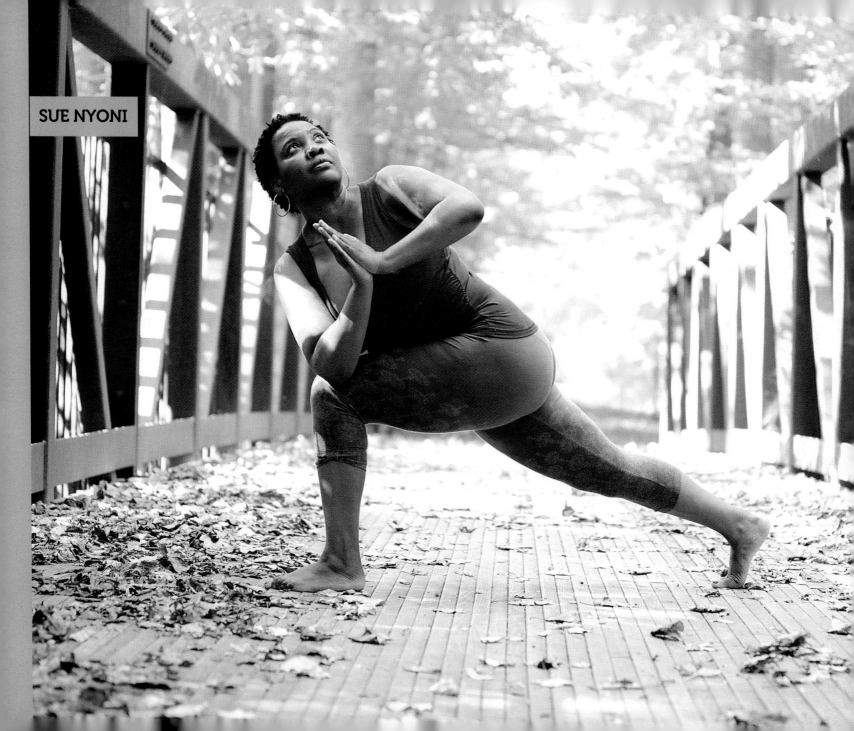

SUE NYONI

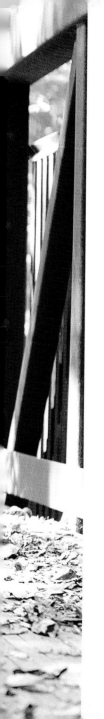

> I disregard the proportions, the measures, the tempo of the ordinary world. I refuse to live in the ordinary world as ordinary women. To enter ordinary relationships. I want ecstasy. I am a neurotic -- in the sense that I live in my world. I will not adjust myself to the world. I am adjusted to myself.
>
> **Anais Nin**

Parivrtta Parshvakonasana (REVOLVING SIDE ANGLE POSE)

Sue's Story...

I have been practicing yoga for about six years. I came to yoga while looking for peace and a way out of the emotional pain I was experiencing in my life. I just wanted a way to live in the world that didn't seem so hard. I was tired of being stressed. I had low self-esteem. I hated my body. I felt unfulfilled and unloved. I really wanted to free myself from the bondage of my own mind.

Yoga has allowed me to develop a healthier relationship with my body. I am learning not to judge and criticize my body for not looking how others think it's supposed to look, or how I've been told it's supposed to look. Instead, as my practice grows and deepens, I am able to see the innate strength and grace in my own body. Rather than constantly criticize it, I now communicate compassion, appreciation, and gratitude to my body. I am also learning to listen to, and be more responsive to what my body needs. It is all about healing my self-image and learning to communicate with my body in ways I had never done before. For me my yoga practice is like daily relationship counseling.

Parivrtta Parsvakonasana is the pose I chose to be photographed in because I love how open it makes me feel. Twisting poses are a real gift to yogis because it allows you to show serious love to your digestive system. Twisting poses are strong, yet graceful. I liken the wringing of the twist to my ability to rid my body of the negative energy that no longer serves me.

I just love the **Nin** quote because this is how I want to live my life. On my own terms! After a lifetime of doing what I thought was expected of me, I am ready to live my life my way.

I **love** my curves because they are God-given, they are mine, and they are beautiful!

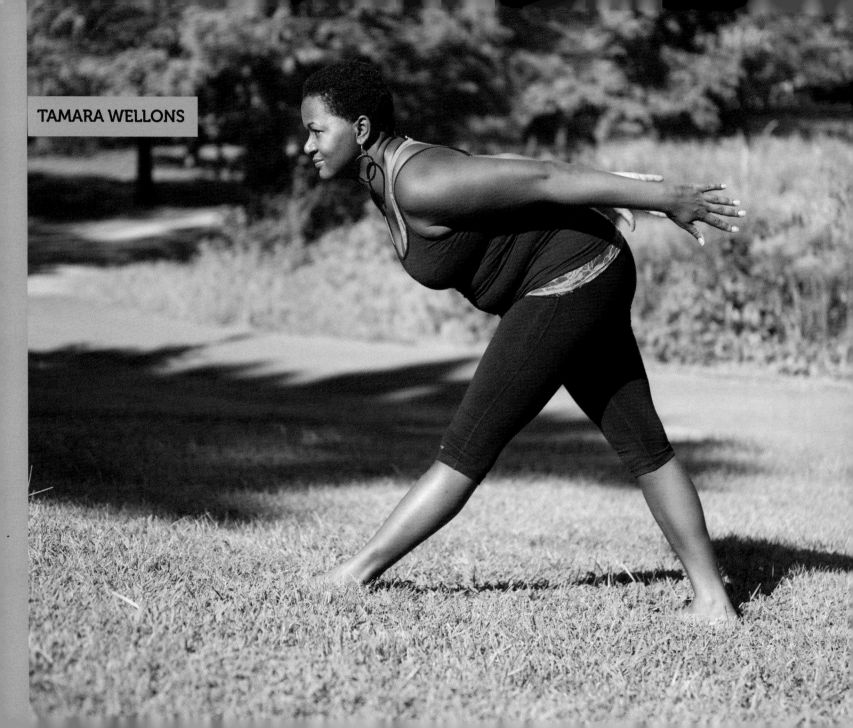

TAMARA WELLONS

Let the Beauty we love be what we do.
Rumi

Parsvottanasana (INTENSE SIDE STRETCH POSE)

Tamara's Story...

I have been practicing yoga for at least eight years off and on. As a child, I did gymnastics, so I was flexible. As an adult, I found the practice of yoga gave me a way to practice my flexibility. I also found yoga to be a useful way to prepare for the birth of my first child.

Parsvottanasana is one of my favorite poses because it invokes grace, strength, and flexibility in life for me. It also gives me a sense of humbleness for the presence of the Most High which is the source of my strength.

Yoga helps me celebrate my curves in many ways. It causes me to pay attention to my curves. I appreciate my legs and body's ability to flex and strengthen as a result. I would tell another curvy woman who wants to start yoga to give it try. Yoga is very calming and gives you a chance to be more in touch with yourself.

One of my favorite quotes is from the poem **Spring Giddiness by Rumi**. I believe that our truest life path unfolds when we do the thing (the beauty) that brings us complete joy.

I **love** my curves because they enhance my personality.

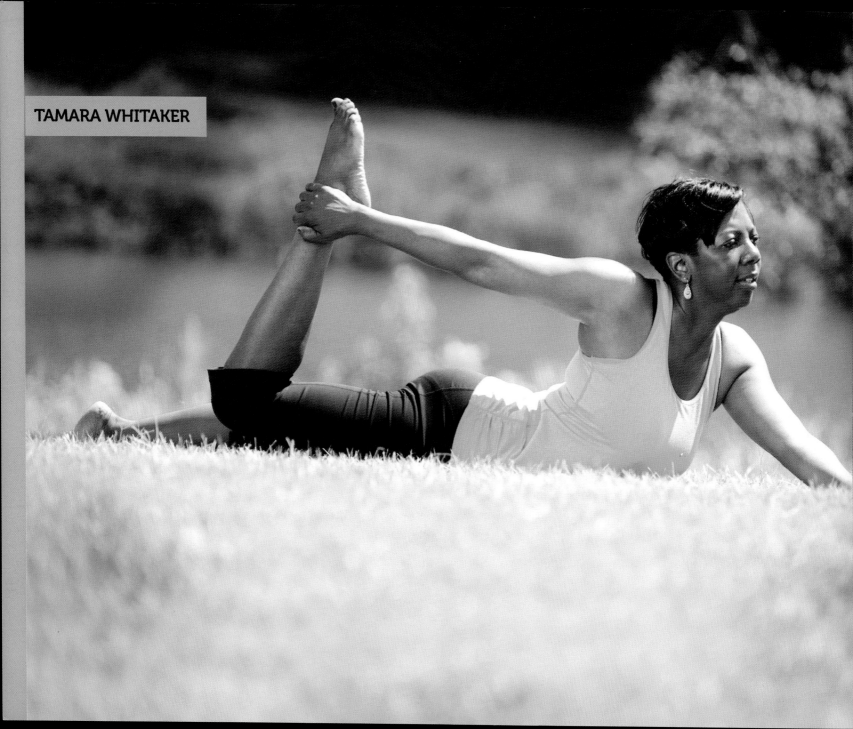

TAMARA WHITAKER

Praise God from whom all Blessings flow.
Thomas Ken

Ardha Dhanurasana (HALF BOW POSE)

Tamara's Story...

I've been practicing yoga off and on for a few years and have been inspired to practice yoga by the desire to stay in shape, and find a form of exercise that emphasizes core strength and stability. I find the workout to be inspiring...the moves, the music, the atmosphere...it all plays into a pleasant but worthwhile experience.

Yoga helps me celebrate and love my body by allowing me to create my own workout. I can choose the intensity of the poses, and practice different levels of intensity all in virtually, the same pose. Yoga makes me feel strong and empowered, and the feeling flows to other aspects of my life.

Ardha Dhanurasana is one of my favorite poses because it forces me to be still, focus, and allow myself time to get into the position. I have found those three lessons to apply to daily life as well as yoga. Since I have been practicing yoga consistently for almost a year now, I have become more focused, and although I wasn't a pessimistic person in the past, I have become more optimistic and my focus continues to be on the positive, on God's blessings, and not on the unfortunate disappointments in life. While the half bow and the bow pose may look simple to the untrained eye, they require stillness, consistent and steady breathing, and gradual positioning. Once in the pose, I feel strong and powerful, energized, and ready to face the day!

I **love** my curves because growing up, I was not proud of the way I looked, and often compared myself to others. As I have gotten older, I appreciate my individual self, and have grown to love the skin I'm in, and curves that I have.

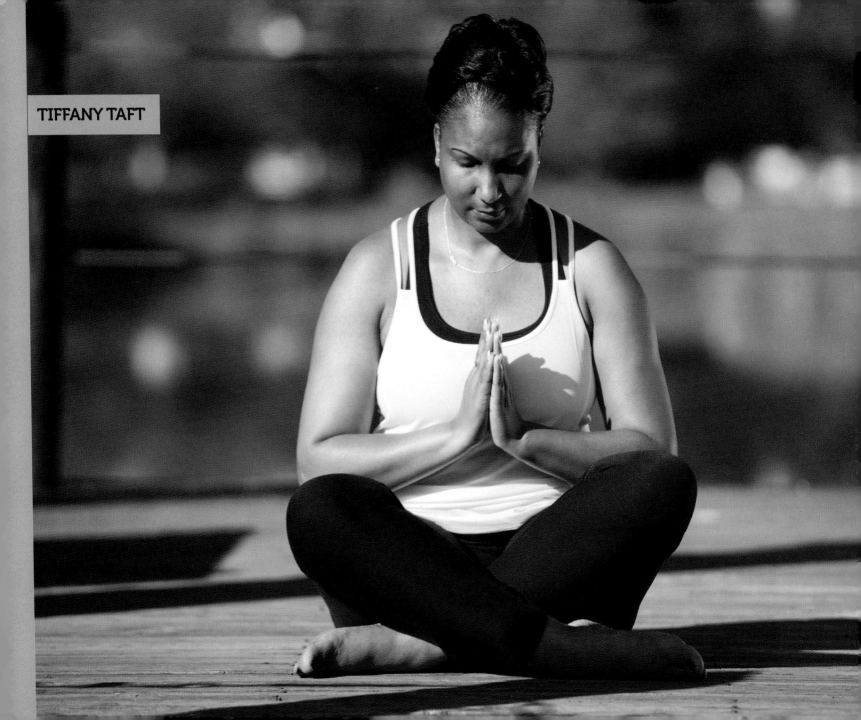

> Be the change.
> **M. K. Gandhi**

Sukhasana (EASY SEATED POSE)

Tiffany's Story...

I started practicing yoga five years ago. At the time, I was seeking greater balance, a more holistic lifestyle, and greater connection to the Source.

Sukhasana is one of my favorite poses as it invokes a sense of calm and peace within my core. It helps ground me and prepares me for the quiet restorative act of meditation. I am able to focus and quiet my mind, while invoking powerful moments of quiet and reflection as I allow myself to just BE STILL. This pose allows me to connect with my breath and really listen to what my body needs, while my mind is open to reflection.

Gandhi's quote speaks to me because I always want to be an inspiration and leave a meaningful message to all that cross my path. I desire and strive to live a life in purpose and service.

I **love** my curves because I am uniquely made and divinely blessed. I embrace my curves in every posture despite the challenges I may feel. I am more aware of just how incredible this body can be and is to me.

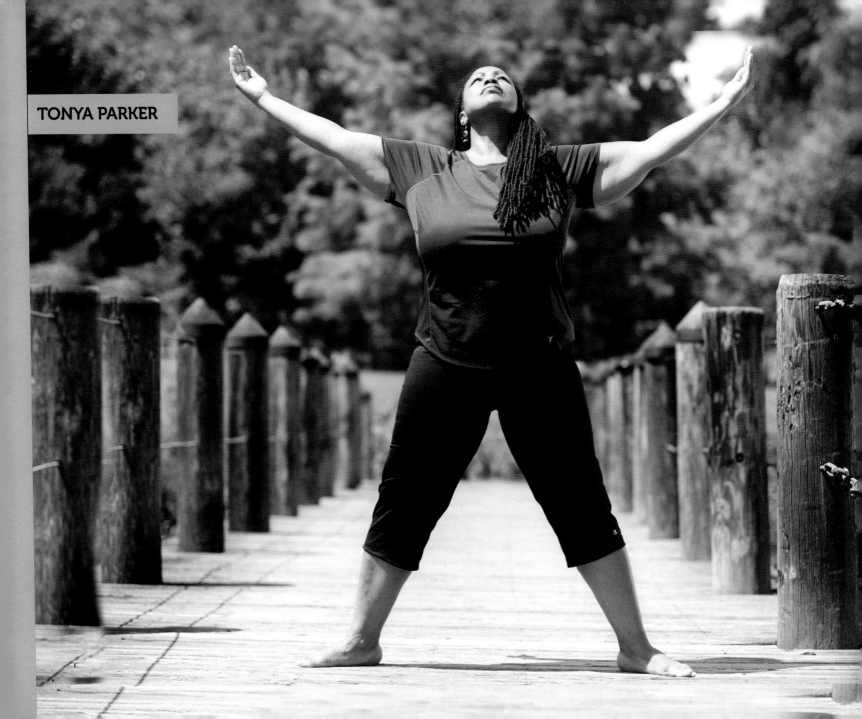

TONYA PARKER

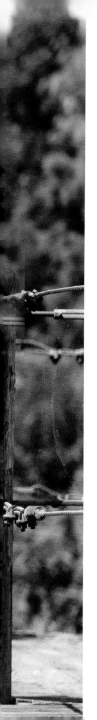

Utthita Tadasana (FIVE-POINTED STAR POSE)

Tonya's Story...

I've been practicing yoga for over 20 years. I was introduced to yoga by a sister graduate student at The College of William & Mary, who came to our office once a week to help us alleviate stress. Yoga resonated with me because as an athlete in high school and college I was disciplined about stretching. I'm 47, and I am committed to making yoga a lifelong practice.

I have always played competitive sports, and yoga has created a wonderful opportunity to refrain from competition with others, and focus on being in tune with my body. I love that as a curvaceous woman, I can still acquire amazing flexibility. I'm grateful for how yoga helped me recover from two low-back surgeries. Even after a hiatus from practice, each time I return to my mat my body responds with ease and effortlessness.

Utthita Tadasana is one of my favorite poses because I love the deceptive simplicity of it. My spine, which has taken a couple of hits, is aligned. My whole body is open to the world, particularly my chest, where my heart chakra resides. Utthita Tadasana symbolizes how I hope I show up in the world—strong, balanced, aligned, and open-hearted—shining brightly like a star!

I love the **Elizabeth Kubler-Ross** quote because it serves as reminder of how I want to show up in the world—allowing my Divine light to always shine and acknowledge the Divine light in all.

I **love** my curves because I love the look and feel of lushness, and I enjoy knowing that I have worked hard to release a good deal of excess weight, but still look like me.

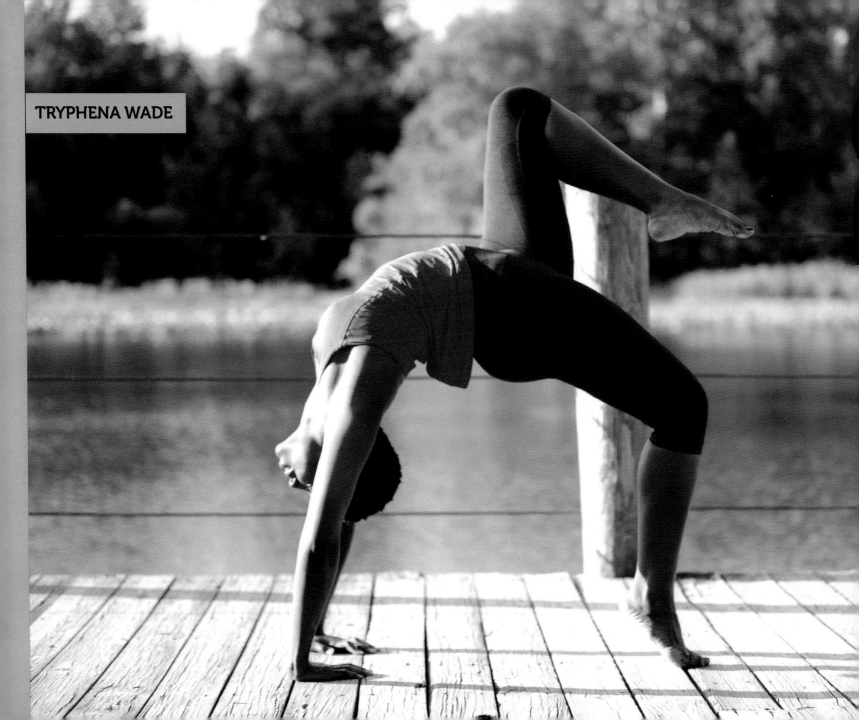

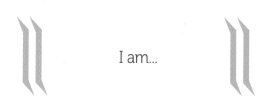

I am...

Urdhva Dhanurasana (WHEEL POSE)

Tryphena's Story...

I've been practicing yoga for about two years. I was required to take a yoga class in college. I didn't understand Sanskrit, and I didn't understand how the asanas would help me. I took classes sporadically, usually at a huge gym in an air conditioned room. I like to sweat when I work out, so taking yoga in a cool room did not appeal to me. Years later I took a hot yoga class. The heat and the sweat and the difficulty of the poses coupled with my ability to do quite a few of them, convinced me to give yoga a second chance.

Through yoga I have experienced increase throughout my life: I have more peace, more strength, and more understanding of how to build and sustain heat within my body. I'm inspired every time I come to my mat. I'm inspired by the poses that come easy and by the more difficult ones.

Urdhva Dhanurasana is one of my favorite poses because I remember a time when it would present itself in my yoga class, and I'd watch everyone else in the class move into it with such ease. Meanwhile, I had no idea where to begin, what to engage, or how to breathe in the pose. I'd try and try with no success. Then one day, it just happened. All my previous attempts had built the strength I needed to actually move into the pose with ease. So for me, this pose represents strength and determination. I feel a freedom and opening in my heart as it rises to the sky.

The phrase, **"I am,"** inspires me to mindful of the words that I speak about myself. It reminds me to use words that are not negative, and to challenge myself in a positive way. I am mindful to say what God would say about me. God is inside of me so whatever He is, I am.

I **love** my curves because they are strong, feminine, and sexy.

YVETTE DAVIS

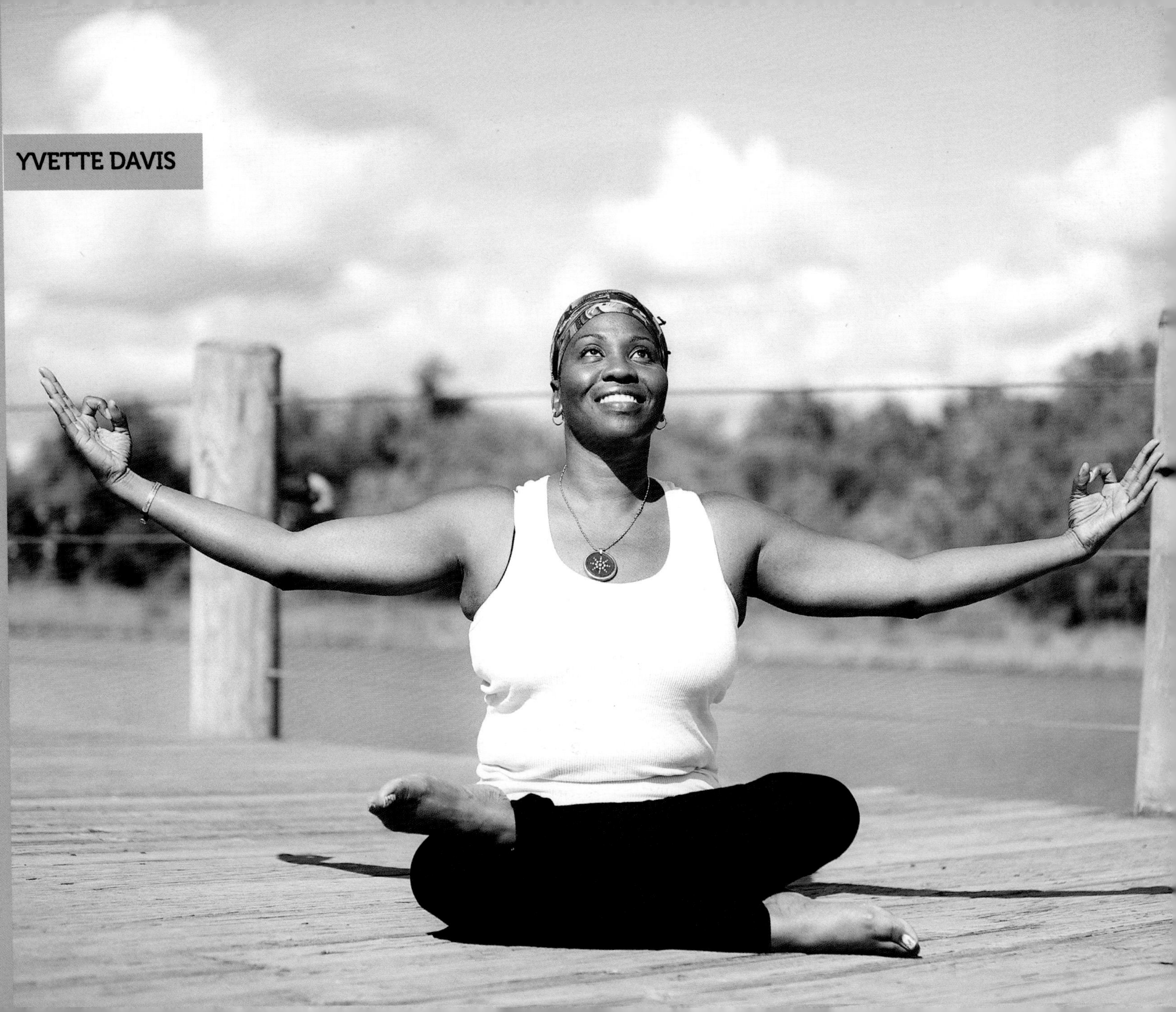

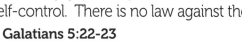

> But the fruit of the Spirit produces love, joy, peace, patience, kindness, goodness, faithfulness, gentleness and self-control. There is no law against these things!
>
> **Galatians 5:22-23**

Agnistambhasana (FIRE LOG POSE)

Yvette's Story...

I've been practicing yoga for over two years and was (and still am) inspired by my 95-year-old cousin, Mrs. Hattie Worthy, who still practices and credits yoga in helping her maintain clarity of mind and mobility.

There are so many ways that yoga is a vital tool in my life. I find that instruction to stay focused in the present works on and off the mat. Also, yoga is an expression of constant love of self in a healthy nurturing way. It also fosters love and support of others, when we share our practice on the mat. By practicing the asanas and reading and learning more about the elements of yoga for your mind, body, and spirit, love begins to express itself visibly in flexibility and weight loss and clarity of mind and spirit—a true expression of love.

Agnistambhasana is one of my favorite poses because it allows me to connect, mind, body, and nature, by the use of sheer gravity, which deepens the expression of the pose by generating energy into the body and allowing the hips to open. I am able to disconnect from my initial apprehension about my knees and begin to relax, flow, and engage the breath in the pose. This allows my body to express itself in the image my mind sees in the present moment and beauty of the experience. Fire log pose is a great way to open the body and release any tension and stress in the body. I encourage others to give it a try, growing into the pose from wherever you are today.

The **Bible scripture** is a gentle reminder for me that each day is a blessing and a gift. I can use my gifts and talents to find my true purpose.

I **love** my curves because they make me uniquely me, and I am grateful for the ability to move and grow in my yoga journey.

Special Thanks to

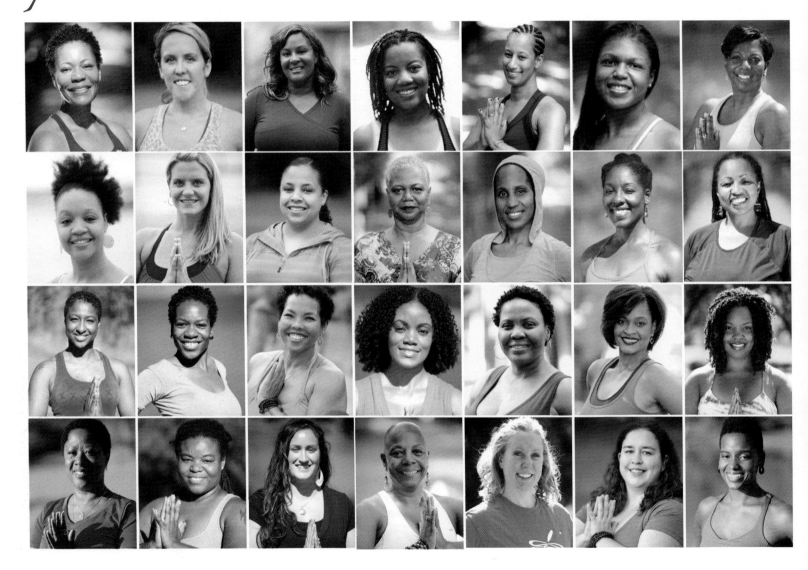

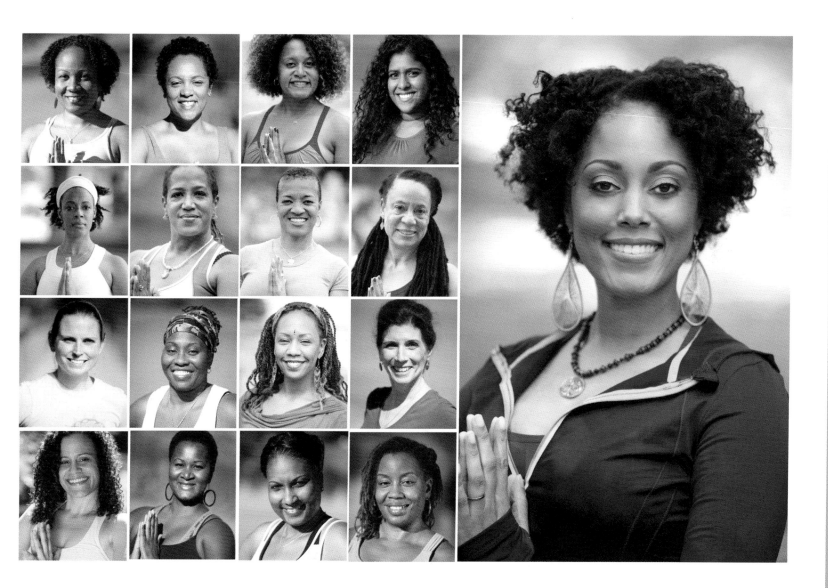

Afterword

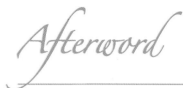

My yoga practice taught me the power of my words and the power of intention. In an effort to stay connected to yoga, both on and off the mat, I created a dedication that I would say to myself while in Savasana. One day, I thought to share it with my class and asked if they would repeat the words after me.

Everyone enjoyed this dedication, and I decided in that moment to make it part of every class I taught, no matter where I was. At the end of one class, I drew a blank and couldn't remember the rest of the dedication. To my surprise, my class continued to recite the words without repeating after me. This touched me deeply and the words still resonate and allow me to carry the energy of strength, courage, flexibility and happiness off the mat and into my world.

As I journey out today,

I will be sure to enjoy every step of the way.

I will walk softly and sweetly with myself, and

Find every reason in the world to love myself, because

I AM LOVED

Index

Curvy Yogini Resources

Yoga Studios

Spiritual Essence Yoga
13100 Brooke Lane
Upper Marlboro, Maryland 20772
www.spiritualessenceyoga.com

Evolution Yoga NC
8411 Mossy Cup Trail
Harrisburg, North Carolina 28075
www.evolutionyoganc.com

Vital Yoga Center
15080 Idlewild Road
Matthews, North Carolina 28104
www.vitalyogacenter.com

Buddha Body Yoga™ with Michael Hayes
39 W. 29th Street, Suite 302
New York, New York 10001
www.buddhabodyoga.com

Harlem Yoga Studio
44 West 125th Street
New York, New York 10027
www.harlemyogastudio.com

PIES Fitness Yoga Studio
374 S Pickett Street
Alexandria, Virginia 22304
www.piesfitnessyoga.com

Lighthouse Yoga Center
4203 Ninth Street NW
Washington, District of Columbia 20011
www.lighthouseyogacenter.com

Ginseng Yoga
2985 Beech Street
San Diego, California 92102
www.ginsengsandiego.com

Gotta Yoga Studio
9539 Pinnacle Drive, Suite. 350
Charlotte, North Carolina 28262
www.gottayogastudio.com

Online Resources

- **Yes Yoga Has Curves:** www.yesyogahascurves.com
- **Yogasteya:** www.yogasteya.com
- **Supportive Yoga:** www.supportiveyoga.com
- **Curvy Yoga:** www.curvyyoga.com
- **Tiina Veer Yoga for Round Bodies:** www.tiinaveer.com
- **Mega Yoga:** www.megayoga.com
- **HeavyWeight Yoga:** www.heavyweightyoga.com
- **Body Positive Yoga:** www.bodypositiveyoga.com
- **Decolonizing Yoga:** www.decolonizingyoga.com
- **Fat Yoga:** www.fatyoga.org

Books

- "Big Yoga: A Simple Guide for Bigger Bodies" by Meera Patricia Kerr
- "MegaYoga: The First Yoga Program for Curvy Women" by Megan Garcia
- "All I Need Is This CHAIR YOGA" by Wilma Carter
- "Health At Every Size: The Surprising Truth About Your Weight" by Linda BaconYasdfasdf

For further information, or to arrange bulk sales or special discounts, please contact:

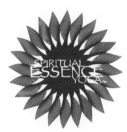

(301) 574-3569 | info@spiritualessenceyoga.com